Transforming Nursing Through Reflective Practice

Transforming Nursing Through Reflective Practice

Edited by
Christopher Johns
Dawn Freshwater

Blackwell
Science

© 1998 by
Blackwell Science Ltd
Editorial Offices:
Osney Mead, Oxford OX2 0EL
25 John Street, London WC1N 2BL
23 Ainslie Place, Edinburgh EH3 6AJ
350 Main Street, Malden
  MA 02148 5018, USA
54 University Street, Carlton
  Victoria 3053, Australia
10, rue Casimir Delavigne
  75006 Paris, France

Other Editorial Offices:

Blackwell Wissenschafts-Verlag GmbH
Kurfürstendamm 57
10707 Berlin, Germany

Blackwell Science KK
MG Kodenmacho Building
7–10 Kodenmacho Nihombashi
Chuo-ku, Tokyo 104, Japan

First published 1998
Reprinted 1998

Set in 10/12 Palatino
by DP Photosetting, Aylesbury, Bucks
Printed and bound in Great Britain by
MPG Books Ltd, Bodmin, Cornwall

The Blackwell Science logo is a trade mark of
Blackwell Science Ltd, registered at the United
Kingdom Trade Marks Registry

DISTRIBUTORS

Marston Book Services Ltd
PO Box 269
Abingdon
Oxon OX14 4YN
(*Orders:* Tel: 01235 465500
        Fax: 01235 465555)

USA
Blackwell Science, Inc.
Commerce Place
350 Main Street
Malden, MA 02148 5018
(*Orders:* Tel: 800 759 6102
            781 388 8250
        Fax: 781 388 8255)

Canada
Login Brothers Book Company
324 Saulteaux Crescent
Winnipeg, Manitoba R3J 3T2
(*Orders:* Tel: 204 837 2987
            204 837 3116)

Australia
Blackwell Science Pty Ltd
54 University Street
Carlton, Victoria 3053
(*Orders:* Tel: 03 9347 0300
        Fax: 03 9347 5001)

A catalogue record for this title
is available from the British Library

ISBN 0-632-04784-4 (pbk.)

Library of Congress
Cataloging-in-Publication Data
Transforming nursing through reflective
  practice/edited by Christopher Johns and
  Dawn Freshwater.
    p. cm.
    Includes bibliographical references and
  index.
    ISBN 0-632-04784-4 (pbk.)
    1. Nursing - Philosophy.
    2. Introspection. 3. Self-knowledge,
  Theory of. I. Johns, Christopher.
  II. Freshwater, Dawn.
    [DNLM: 1. Nursing.   WY 16 T772 1998]
  RT84.5.T73   1998
  610.73 - dc21
  DNLM/DLC
  for Library of Congress   97-31578
                                          CIP

For practitioners everywhere who care

Contents

Preface   ix
Acknowledgement   xi
List of Contributors   xii

1   Opening the Doors of Perception   1
   Christopher Johns

2   Beyond Expertise: Reflective and Reflexive Nursing Practice   21
   Gary Rolfe

3   Doing the Right Thing: Customary vs Reflective Morality
   in Nursing Practice   32
   Lucie Ferrell

4   Nursing as Caring Through the Reflective Lens   43
   Anne Boykin

5   Voice as a Metaphor for Transformation Through Reflection   51
   Christopher Johns and Helen Hardy

6   Unfolding the Conditions where the Transformative
   Potential of Guided Reflection (Clinical Supervision) might
   Flourish or Flounder   62
   Christopher Johns and Brendan McCormack

7   Illuminating the Transformative Potential of
   Guided Reflection   78
   Christopher Johns

8   Transforming Nursing Through Reflective Practice   91
   Judy Lumby

9 Exploration of the Empowering Potential of Clinical
   Supervision, Reflection and Action Research   104
   Carolyn Moore and Julia Carter

10 Understanding the Nature of Nursing Through Reflection:
   a Case Study Approach   119
   Iain Graham

11 Locating a Phenomenological Perspective of Reflective
   Nursing and Midwifery Practice by Contrasting Interpretive
   and Critical Reflection   134
   Bev Taylor

12 Reflection and Expert Nursing Knowledge   151
   Jane Glaze

13 Reflective Practice – a Way to the Patient's World and
   Caring, the Core of Nursing   161
   Tina Nordman, Anne Kasén and Katie Eriksson

14 The Philosopher's Stone   177
   Dawn Freshwater

15 The Reflective Journey Begins a Spiritual Journey   185
   Stephen Wright

16 The Supervisor's Story: from Expert to Novice   194
   Jan Bailey

17 The Rocky Road to Reflection   206
   Myra Davis

18 A Meta-reflection on Reflective Practice and Caring Theory   214
   Jean Watson

Index   221

Preface

This book is the story of a group of people who came together through the experience of the Third Reflective Practice conference that took place in July 1996 at Robinson College, Cambridge. The contributions within this book have been developed from conference papers focused around the theme: 'Transformation of Nursing through Reflective Practice'. The contributions by Bev Taylor 'Chapter 11' and Christopher Johns 'Chapter 7' were invited to add a further dimension to this story. If the book is the whole story, then each chapter is a story within this story. Within each of these contributions are the stories of nurses, patients, teachers, practitioners, people, human beings. As the group bonded and the stories unfolded, each contribution revealed its own unique essence of humanness. Yet the threads of connectedness are so obvious that they are almost invisible; seamless. This story itself is, part of a larger, universal story as the individuals within this story were transformed through the collective experience of the conference. Without doubt, the conference was remarkable in realising the potential of nursing as caring – healing through reflection, as a collective expanding consciousness. We ask you to reflect as you read this book, to engage with and relate to the writers' stories from a personal perspective. The book is not offered as a prescription or an explanation – that would be counter to the spirit of reflection – it is offered as a source of wisdom to guide you and to help you make sense of your own experience of reflection and transformation.

To design your future, visualize where you want to be, and then build the bridge from your present, to that place. Your vision becomes your destiny, and your bridge becomes your path. Assure your bridge is strong with a well-defined plan. Flow with time but be present with each moment ... like all the winged, in order to transcend, we too, must be in movement. We must vibrate. Truth after truth after truth reveals itself at each fluttering of our spiritual wings. Like the gradual shading of blue to green, we become, we live the transformations. It is as though we are in a cocoon within a cocoon, within a cocoon. The more truth we experience, the more we are set free in colourful flight. Always in movement, the different levels of consciousness we experience lead us to the next level. This is how we come to soar!

Blackwolf and Gina Jones

It is tempting to 'explain' why we have chosen to include these words by Blackwolf and Gina Jones in the Preface. We feel this temptation because we live in a world that is short of imagination; a world that has been dominated by rational thinking where all things can be explained given time. A world short of imagination is also a world short of creativity, short of vision and short of soul. We feel that Blackwolf and Gina Jones give this book the direction in which we hope to travel – a stimulating and inquisitive journey into higher levels of consciousness, where we as nurses can move towards becoming the kinds of people we want to be, fulfilling our therapeutic destiny and enabling those with whom we work with to fulfil theirs. To quote Thomas Beckett (1969):

> 'To be capable of helping others to become all they are capable of becoming we must first fulfil that commitment to ourselves.'

We feel that reflection offers a path along which to make this journey of mutual growth and becoming. Reflection gives us wings to soar as we emerge from our cocoons.

In view of the fact that the great majority of nurses are women, the pronouns 'she' and 'her' will be used throughout this book. This measure has been taken for simplicity and is in no way intended to offend or alienate our male colleagues.

Christopher Johns and *Dawn Freshwater*

References

Beckett, T. (1969) A candidate's reflections on the supervisory process. *Contemporary Psychoanalysis*, 5, 169–179.
Jones, R. Blackwolf & Jones, G. (1996) *Earth Dance Drum*. Commune-E-Key Publishing, Salt Lake City.

Acknowledgement

We offer our thanks to all those who gave their help and support in bringing this book into being, particularly Sarah-Kate Powell at Blackwell Science.

List of Contributors

Jan Bailey BA(Hons), PGDipEd, PGDip Advanced Health Care Practice, RMN, RNT
Senior Lecturer, Faculty of Health Care and Social Studies, University of Luton

Anne Boykin PhD, RN, BSN, MN
Dean and Professor, Florida Atlantic University, College of Nursing, Boca Raton, Florida

Julia Carter RGN
Senior Staff Nurse, Medical Unit, Leicester General Hospital NHS Trust

Myra Davies RGN, BA(Hons)
Matron, The Sue Ryder Foundation, St Johns Palliative Care Home, Moggerhanger, Bedfordshire

Katie Eriksson PhD, RN
Professor in Caring Science, Department of Caring Science, Åbo Akademi University, Vasa, Finland, and Professor in Nursing Science, Department of Primary Healthcare, University of Helsinki, Finland

Lucie Ferrell RH, PhD
Associate Professor, Department of Nursing, Augsburg College, Minneapolis, Minnesota, USA

Dawn Freshwater BA(Hons), RGN, RNT, Dip Couns, Dip EHPNLP, FETC
Senior Lecturer in Nursing Studies, Homerton College, Cambridge School of Health Studies

Jane Glaze RN, BSc, PhD
Senior Lecturer, School of Nursing, University of Wolverhampton

Iain Graham MEd, MSc, BSc, RN
Head of Department of Nursing, Midwifery and Health Visiting, Institute of Health and Community Studies, Bournemouth University

Helen Hardy BA, RGN
Staff Nurse, Adolescent Unit, Royal National Orthopaedic Hospital, Stanmore, Middlesex

Christopher Johns MN, PhD, RGN, RMN
Reader in Advanced Nursing Practice, Faculty of Health Care and Social Studies, University of Luton

Anne Kasén MNSc, RN
Doctoral student, Department of Caring Science, Åbo Akademi University, Vasa, Finland

Judy Lumby RN, PhD, MHPEd, BA, FRCNA, FRCN
Chair of Surgical Nursing, Faculty of Nursing, The University of Sydney, and Concord Repatriation General Hospital, Australia

Brendan McCormack BSc (Hons) Nursing, DPSN, PGCEA, RNT, RGN, RMN
Royal College of Nursing Institute and Oxfordshire Community Trust, Radcliffe Infirmary, Oxford, and Programme Director (Community Hospitals & Gerontological Nursing)

Carolyn Moore RGN, DipN, MSc
Practice Development Nurse Manager, Royal Cornwall Hospitals Trust (Treliske), Truro, Cornwall

Tina Nordman MNSc, RN
Doctoral Student, Department of Caring Science, Åbo Akademi University, Vasa, Finland

Gary Rolfe BSc, RMN, MA, PGCEA, PhD
Principal Lecturer, University of Portsmouth, School of Health Studies, St James' Hospital, Portsmouth

Bev Taylor RN, RM, MEd, PhD
Professor, School of Nursing and Health Care Practices, Southern Cross University, New South Wales, Australia

Jean Watson RN, PhD, FAAN
Distinguished Professor of Nursing and Director, Center for Human Caring, University of Colorado Health Sciences Center, Denver, Colorado, USA

Stephen Wright MBE, RGN, DipN, RCNT, DANS, RNT, MSc, MHSM, FRCN
Director of The European Nursing Development Agency Ltd (TENDA), Cumbria, and Visiting Professor of Nursing at the University of Southampton

Chapter 1
Opening the Doors of Perception

Christopher Johns

Introduction

Reflective practice is topical. Any nursing or educational journal seems to contain at least one paper that talks about reflection. Why is this? The influence of Patricia Benner must be acknowledged in focusing attention on the nature of expertise, and most significantly, how Benner (1984) drew on the Dreyfus and the Dreyfus model of skill acquisition to consider the way the expert practitioner makes decisions and takes action in practice situations. The expert responds intuitively to situations, responding to the whole situation. This is in contrast with the novice who is reliant on breaking down situations into stages within a linear decision-making process. Readers may recognise such a process in the nursing process, that characteristically breaks down situations into 'assessment', 'problem', 'planning', 'action' and 'evaluation'. It quickly becomes apparent that such models are inappropriate for the 'expert' practitioner simply because 'experts' do not think like this. Such models may also be educationally inappropriate for less expert practitioners as they learn to become increasingly expert.

Benner notes that intuition is based on a deep understanding of the situation. This knowing is embodied within self. It is a holistic knowing that is able to grasp the meaning of the whole situation in a moment and respond appropriately. Dreyfus and Dreyfus recognised that in responding intuitively to the situation, the expert practitioner draws on past concrete experience to inform this response. This is not a deliberative searching through the memory but the very nature of tacit knowing. By this I mean that it is the knowing embodied within the practitioner that is difficult to articulate. As Schön (1983) has noted, the knowing is in our doing. If I was to watch an expert practitioner respond to a distressed patient I would be observing this tacit knowing. The 'expertness' would be apparent in the performance. If I was to ask the practitioner afterwards to talk me through the way she responded she might struggle to articulate quite how she had done this. She might say something like 'Well, I just responded to her. She needed support at this time'. Intuition is the active expression of this tacit knowing. Yet it is a type of knowing that has not been easily accepted in a world dominated by rational thinking. I am sure many readers of this book will remember situations when they knew something intuitively only to be scorned for a lack of observable evidence. Visinstainer (1986) noted that:

> 'Even when nurses govern their own practice, they succumb to the belief that the "soft stuff" such as feelings and beliefs and support are not quite as substantive as the hard data from laboratory reports and sophisticated monitoring.' (p. 37)

Instead of honouring our intuition we have come to doubt it. Practitioners have internalised this lack of worth in their intuitions and clinical or educational processes have not focused on developing intuition – at least until now. Reflection gives access to past concrete experience in order to develop the reservoir of tacit knowing. Reflective practice feels like a new dawn, as if the curtain of doubt has been thrown aside to display a new horizon of opportunity towards realising nursing's therapeutic potential.

Reflective practice

Yet what is reflective practice? It seems an academic pastime to try and define exactly what it is. This is, of course, the legacy of rational thought – to know the thing in itself. Hence the predilection for definition – to know what reflective practice is so it can be controlled and manipulated towards certain ends. When I commenced using reflection within practice with primary nurses at Burford hospital in 1989, I simply asked them to talk about 'experiences' in their everyday practice which they felt were significant for whatever reasons. These were usually infused with a degree of doubt, anxiety, distress, unresolved conflict, and occasionally satisfaction. I suggested that it might be helpful to write about these experiences within a journal. The definitions of reflection did not help this process. For example, Boyd and Fales (1983) define reflection as being:

> 'The process of creating and clarifying the meaning of experience in terms of self in relation to both self and the world. The outcome of this process is changed conceptual perspectives.' (p. 101)

In other words, through reflection the practitioner may come to see the world differently, and based on these new insights may come to act differently as a changed person. Other theorists, such as Mezirow (1981) and Boud, *et al.* (1985) say similar things. Street (1992) drew the conclusion from her critical ethnography of nursing practice that:

> 'The confrontation with experience through reflection and of the meanings and assumptions which surround it, can form a foundation

upon which to make choices about future actions based on chosen value systems and new ways of thinking about and understanding nursing practice.' (p. 16)

Gary Rolfe in Chapter 2 offers some significant insights into the relationship between reflection-in-action and intuition, within the context of expertise. In considering the relationship between intuition and habitual practice, Gary suggests that intuition is a kind of conscious mindlessness. However, the expert practitioner does respond to situations appropriately and with great skill, which suggests intuition is a highly sophisticated and holistic processing of information, an issue developed by Dawn Freshwater in Chapter 14.

Perhaps the person who simply responds in a habitual way can never be described as an expert because they fail to consider the unique context of the situation and merely fall back on known ways of responding. Related to this, it is necessary to challenge the idea of 'irrational intuition'.

Intuition is the manifestation of tacit knowledge, a knowing that is deeply embodied but unable to be expressed in rational ways. Gary draws on a number of theorists to support his position but it is pertinent to challenge the agendas of commendators such as Brook and Champion, Elstein and Bordage, and Andrews. Are they simply people who are locked into rational ways of thinking that must inherently reject the validity of intuition unless it can be ultimately explained in rational ways? A reflection of what counts as valid knowledge is a legacy of scientific rationalism. Our view is that knowing in practice is a constructed knowledge – a subjective, holistic and contextual knowing that has been appropriately informed by empirical science and theory. This is the most significant type of knowledge because it is the knowledge used in practice, and is used either in deliberative rational ways or in intuitive ways as appropriate, to best respond to the unfolding clinical moment.

My careful recording of the dialogue that took place between myself and practitioners within the first two years of guided reflection (1989–1991 as part of my doctoral study (Johns 1997c)) enabled me to look back and analyse the patterns of interaction. From this analysis I constructed the model of structured reflection (MSR) with the intention of enabling the practitioner to 'know' what it meant to reflect (Fig. 1.1). Patterns of certain questions emerged that seemed significant in helping a practitioner explore the meaning of experience in ways that meant experience could be learnt from. The MSR is a heuristic device to enable practitioners to penetrate the essence of reflection-on-experience. It offers an answer to the question: 'How do I reflect?' By heuristic I mean that the MSR does not intend to prescribe how the practitioner *should* reflect. In time, through using the model in a concrete way, the practitioner will internalise and transcend the model, fusing the cues into her own reflective lens. This would then give structure to reflective writing. Over time the MSR has reflexively developed through reflection on its use.

Write a description of the experience.
What are the significant issues I need to pay attention to? (This cue has been re-inserted into the 10th edition)

Reflective cues:

Aesthetics	What was I trying to achieve?
	Why did I respond as I did?
	What were the consequences of that for:
	• the patient?
	• others?
	• myself?
	How was this person(s) feeling?
	How did I know this?
Personal	How did I feel in this situation?
	What internal factors were influencing me?
Ethics	How did my actions match with my beliefs?
	What factors made me act in incongruent ways?
Empirics	What knowledge did or should have informed me?
Reflexivity	How does this connect with previous experiences?
	Could I handle this better in similar situations?
	What would the consequences be of alternative actions for:
	• the patient?
	• others?
	• myself?
	How do I *now* feel about this experience?
	Can I support myself and others better as a consequence?
	Has this changed my ways of knowing?

Fig. 1.1   Model of structured reflection/10a

I framed the reflective cues within Strauss and Corbin's 'paradigm' model for grounded theory (Strauss & Corbin 1990). The 'paradigm' model intended to enable the grounded theory researcher to think systematically about complex data at an appropriate level of precision and density. The influence of this model led me initially to encourage the practitioner to split 'description' of the experience into phenomenon, causal and context parts (Johns 1994a). However, it soon became clear that this splitting into parts interfered with practitioners telling their stories. The causal and contextual factors were properly given attention as factors that influenced the practitioners' actions. The significance of creating opportunity for practitioners to tell their stories is captured by Mishler (1986), who noted:

'Telling stories is a significant way for individuals to give meaning to and express their understanding of their experience.' (p. 75)

The practitioner is encouraged to tell her story. Anne Boykin in Chapter 4 makes the connections between storytelling and reflection, expressing the experience of revealing humanness through an oral tradition. Having told her story the practitioner is encouraged to identify what is significant within the story, to begin to focus the reflective effort. The cues reflect cognitive, affective and temporal aspects of experience.

Ways of knowing

The tenth edition of the MSR reorganised the reflective cues to focus the practitioner on the fundamental ways of knowing, as identified by Barbara Carper (1978) and Johns (1995). Through reflection, the practitioner can begin to understand the way the personal, ethical, and empiric ways of knowing have informed the aesthetic response (Fig. 1.2).

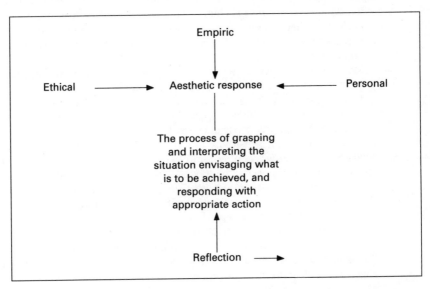

Fig. 1.2 The inter-relation within Carper's fundamental ways of knowing in nursing.

These ways of knowing offer a comprehensive and valid framework for viewing learning through reflection. When a practitioner tells her story, she is sharing a description of the 'aesthetic response'. Consider the following story I wrote in my reflective journal following a shift one morning in a hospice:

Melissa

10.30 – I was working with Susan who was 'in charge' of the shift. We went to inform Stephanie, another staff nurse, that the husband of one of her patients wanted to talk with the doctor. Stephanie was in the room with Melissa, another patient. We hovered outside the room. After a few minutes Stephanie opened the door and Susan informed her of the husband's request.

Stephanie took this opportunity to get Susan to check some 'oromorph' for Melissa. She was in considerable distress with lower back pain. She had spinal cord compression due to spinal metastases from a primary sarcoma that had required her left leg to be amputated. She had the pain because she had been asleep and had woken late. Effectively she had missed a dose. Her breakfast also arrived. I went in and said 'hello'. I felt a need to be involved on some clinical level this morning. Melissa burst into tears, but apologised immediately for her tears, saying 'you've caught me at a tearful moment' and trying hard not to cry. She informed me that she had this pain which had brought down her defences. She said she was not crying for herself but for her family and friends left behind. She was feeling their pain for them. She wanted it to be all right for them and she didn't know how to make it all right for them.

I was conscious of a furious scrabble inside me in order to respond appropriately, to tune into this woman, to make sense of her distress that rippled across the surface of her being. What would be the right words to say? What would I be trying to achieve? To reassure her? To reassure myself? To acknowledge her feelings as reasonable? To acknowledge her need to 'fix-it' for others? My difficulty was in not knowing her – not being able to interpret what she wanted.

My scrabble inside was an unscrambling of this information to appraise her pattern manifestation and to help her find meaning in this experience in ways which would mean she could take control of her life; to grow through this crisis, as a process of expanding consciousness – Margaret Newman's theory of health as expanding consciousness. I was conscious of my internal dialogue, conscious of my sensitivity to self synchronising with my sensitivity to Melissa, my empathy; yet how could I know what this woman was feeling as she contemplated her death and the impact of her death on others? I remembered the words from *Final Gifts* (Kelley & Callanan 1992), how the dying person needs to reassure herself that those being left behind could manage – a theoretical framework to pin the issues within.

I didn't know what to say to Melissa, beyond: 'I can see this is hard for you right now'; in other words acknowledging the feeling and her task, whilst trying hard to focus my concern to let her know I cared for her. And then my role became clear: to simply be there for her and feel conscious of establishing a dialogue with her. My task was to get onto her wave-length, to tune into who she was – and yet I knew nothing about her. Hence my struggling, and yet within just a few minutes I knew enough about who she was at that time to begin this caring dance with her.

Melissa said to sit down, which I did – an acknowledgement of acceptance from her. She grimaced with the pain as she received her 'oromorph'. I stayed with her for a further 10 minutes. She said she was usually all right, that in fact she had a strong spiritual coping. She was approaching her death from this almost objective spiritual perspective which gave her comfort. In moments of weakness, when the pain broke through, her defences were shredded, exposing her vulnerability and the fragility of her spiritual coping. I could see I could help her on this level.

I felt calm inside now. I felt for this brave woman with her fragile smile who had suffered so much and whose life was in crisis in other ways with the breakdown of her marriage and her need to move home at this time. I took her hand as I said goodbye, and said it was good to meet her. She reciprocated.

Later when I went with Susan and the doctor on 'the round', she told them about how weepy she had been and how this young man had been there with her, comforting her. She smiled at me and I knew we had connected. I was reassured that I had helped her and felt warm towards her. I needed this warmth from her. In the midst of suffering, joy can be found through the caring–healing dance.

My aesthetic response to the situation was the way I grasped and interpreted what was happening, whilst trying to envisage what Melissa needed at this time, and how I responded within the unfolding situation. Meeting Melissa for the first time under these circumstances made this a very tough situation for me to respond to adequately. Hence it is a story of my struggle to know Melissa. I drew on my past experience and empathy in my effort to 'tune into' Melissa's wavelength, to connect with her.

The 'personal' aspect reflects who I am as a person, the extent of my concern for Melissa, the way I can manage my own concerns so they do not interfere with seeing Melissa's concerns – the way I manage my anxiety within the situation. The 'ethical' is concerned with doing the right thing. For example, should I have even gone into her room at this time because I had a need to say 'hello'? The 'empiric' relates to knowledge I drew on to inform my understanding and response within the situation.

Carper's ways of knowing are not, in themselves, a model for facilitating reflection. Indeed, the ways of knowing were inadequate because knowing always needs to be contextualised as a historical and cultural process (White 1995). Hence I constructed a fifth way of knowing, which I labelled 'reflexivity' to account for this. Reflexivity acknowledges that 'an experience' is not an isolated moment but part of a continuous flow of experience over spatial and temporal time. As such, 'an experience' is always a reflection of past experience that anticipates future experience. Indeed this is the fundamental learning process, of making sense of the present in terms of the past, with a view towards the future. This is important to understand in the way people construct learning opportunity based on reflection within curriculum and within clinical supervision. This understanding also deals with criticism of reflection as being retrospective (Greenwood 1993), or distorted by hindsight (Reece Jones 1995), or by limitations of memory recall (Newell 1992). It is not the accuracy of reflection that is significant but the meaning the practitioner gives to the situation. That the meaning may be distorted is irrelevant because it is distorted for reasons that are themselves important to understand. That is why reflection always needs to be guided.

Understanding factors that influence ways of responding

Many practitioners have published accounts of reflection using the MSR. Karen Elcock (1997) noted I had omitted the cue question – 'what external factors influenced by decision making and actions?' – from the 10th edition. There are two schools of thought on the idea that 'things' exist outside us that determine how we might act within any situation. Street (1992) exemplifies this position. She states:

'A great many actions that we perform are not the result of conscious knowledge or choice, but are caused by social conditions over which we have no control.' (p. 7)

This is a very passive position. In contrast Cox *et al.* (1991) note that:

'By reflecting in a committed way we may come to see that many of our deepest beliefs about our nursing world may be contradicted in the ways we think and act; and we may discover that it is not through external forces unrelated to ourselves that we are prevented from meeting our ideals but through the way that we perceived ourselves, our actions, and our worlds.' (p. 387)

In other words, barriers only exist within the practitioner. These barriers are projected onto the external situation and acted upon as if outside the practitioner. They are *perceived* as barriers because they lead the practitioner to act in certain ways.

Such factors can be arranged within a grid to help the practitioner to consider the reflective cue within the MSR – 'What internal factors were influencing me?' (Fig. 1.3). The identified factors are commonly perceived barriers that have been evident within practitioners' shared experiences. The value of stating these within the grid is to draw the practitioner's attention to them in the context of the particular experience.

Expectations from self: • obligation/duty • conscience • beliefs/values	Negative attitude towards the patient/family?	Expectations from others: • in what way?
Normal practice – felt I had to conform to a certain action	**What factors influenced my actions?**	Loyalty to staff versus loyalty to patient/family?
Fear of sanction?	Time/priorities?	Anxious about ensuing conflict?

Fig. 1.3   Grid for considering 'What factors influenced my actions?' (Model of structured reflection, 10th edition, Johns 1997a).

This grid is similar in concept to the 'ethical mapping grid' I constructed to help practitioners consider the reflective cue, 'How did my actions match with my beliefs?' (Figure 1.4) (Johns 1997b). Ethical mapping intends to help practitioners 'see' the various contextual factors within any ethical decision. At each point within this 'map', the practitioner is challenged to understand and balance the dynamics towards making the 'right' decision within the particular circumstance by drawing attention to different people's perspectives and factors that

Patient's/family's perspective	*Authority to act?*	The doctor's perspective
Conflict of values?	**The situation/ dilemma**	*Ethical principles?*
The nurses' perspective	*Power relationships?*	The organisation's perspective

Fig. 1.4 Grid for considering 'How did my actions match with my beliefs?' (Model of structured reflection, 10th edition, Johns 1997b).

influence decision-making. Lucie Ferrell (Chapter 3) offers a model of ethical reasoning based on reflection. She posits that ethics are not something to apply but to understand within the situation; that what is right can only be known within the situation.

The factors identified within these two grids reflect significant issues that have emerged from analysing practitioners' shared experiences over time. They help to expose and understand the factors that contribute to the nature of contradiction between desirable practice and actual practice. Contradiction is the essential learning opportunity within reflection. Based on this understanding I have defined reflection as:

> 'Reflection-on-experience is a window for practitioners to look inside and know who they are as they strive towards understanding and realising the meaning of desirable work in their everyday practices. The practitioner must expose, confront and understand the contradictions, within their practice, between what is practised and what is desirable. It is the conflict of contradiction and the commitment to achieve desirable work that empowers the practitioner to take action to appropriately resolve these contradictions.' (Johns 1996).

Knowing desirable practice

The MSR reflective cue – 'What was I trying to achieve?' – intends to help the practitioner clarify and find meaning in her beliefs and values and to understand the factors that inhibit these becoming a lived reality. It is significant to ask what is understood as 'desirable practice', in order to give meaning to the idea of transformation. Within her reflections, Helen Hardy (Chapter 5) discusses the significance of 'connected relationships' in terms of her belief that nursing is fundamentally patient-centred. Few nurses, if any, would disagree with this belief. Yet in practice, many nurses continue to reduce the patient to the status of a 'medical label' because they remain in the shadow of a dominant and pervasive medical model. Figure 1.5 is a good illustration of contradiction.

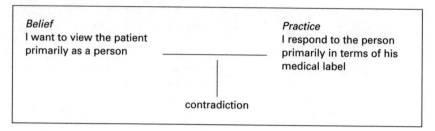

Fig. 1.5   Illustration of contradiction in attitude to patient.

Helen's learning effort through reflection is to resolve this contradiction. She illustrates how she draws on extant theory to help her make sense of her experience and to inform and expand her empathic viewing lens. The MSR poses the reflective cue, 'What information did or should have informed my actions?' The reflective practitioner always needs to interpret extant theory for its relevance and usefulness within the particular situation. In doing so the reflective practitioner inherently rejects the idea that theory exists to predict or prescribe clinical practice. This rejection is based in the belief that each encounter between the nurse and the patient is a unique human encounter.

Few nurses would disagree that this is true. Understanding this reinforces the absurdity of the nursing process in 'planning care'. Indeed, to plan care threatens to reduce the patient to some medically defined object to be manipulated towards certain treatment norms. The nursing process approach also encourages stereotyped and unimaginative approaches, and conformity to normal practice. From a reflective perspective, the practitioner needs to grasp and interpret the meaning of this situation whilst in it, and based on this understanding and envisaging with the patient what needs to be achieved, to respond appropriately. The situation cannot be predicted, although the practitioner may have a deep understanding of similar situations because of her previous experiences informed by relevant theory.

Helen works as a staff nurse on an adolescent orthopaedic ward. The experiences she used within Chapter 5 were initially part of an assignment she completed as part of the requirement of undertaking the 'Becoming a reflective and effective practitioner' [ENB A29] course. The assignment challenged her to look back and make sense of her learning through reflection-on-experience in ways that demonstrated her reflexive growth or illuminated barriers that limited that achievement. Helen and I plot the growth of her practice through the stages of 'developing voice' using the work of Belenky *et al.* (1986). Of course, developing voice is not the same as transformation. Transformation is only known through action. Yet voice is a metaphor that marks the growth of transformation, reflected in the way Helen became able to talk differently about herself and her practice through the reflective medium.

This is an important contribution to the book because Helen is an ordinary nurse working on an ordinary ward. And yet the potential for change of self and practice is so vivid. It exists within every nurse. Helen, like most nurses, like most people, has the capacity to be extra-ordinary. Indeed Helen becomes extraordinary. Her story merely highlights how socialisation processes had squashed or contained this caring potential in Helen. She was fortunate to be exposed to a powerful reflective learning milieu over 30 weeks, that created the transformative moment. The challenge is to create such opportunity as routine, if nurses and nursing can be transformed to reach their therapeutic destiny as a caring–healing power for people.

Seeing beyond self

Helen Hardy was guided to learn through reflection. In a recent guided reflection session I explored with a practitioner, with whom I had been working for two years, the extent to which she still felt she needed guidance. I challenged her whether she was now able to supervise herself. In doing so I asked her to monitor her ability to self-challenge along the following continuum:

| need to be | | can adequately |
| challenged | ——————————————⌐—— | self-challenge |

I then asked her to monitor the extent she now felt she 'knew herself':

still do not		know myself
know self		well enough
well enough	——————————————⌐——	now

Not surprisingly the two perceptions matched each other. The gap between the mark and the end of the line symbolised the extent that she needed help to 'see beyond herself'. Although she had internalised reflection and responsibility to ensure and monitor her own effective-ness, she felt she would still struggle to see beyond her normal ways of viewing and responding to practice. I suggested she used the MSR deliberately over the three weeks before our next session so we could see the extent that she could or could not 'see beyond herself' in terms of factors that influenced her actions within specific situations.

Elcock (1997) noted that as an occasional yet regular visitor to the cardiology ward, she could see 'normal practice' for its impact on achieving therapeutic nursing more easily than the staff embedded within the normal practice of the ward. To again quote Cox *et al.*:

'Reflection in isolation is difficult to sustain because of the difficulty in surfacing and transcending what may be our own distorted self understanding, asking ourselves difficult, often self-exposing ques-tions, facing the difficult answers to such questions, and perhaps, most particularly keeping our vision directed towards new possibi-lities for understanding and action.' (p. 385)

Understanding this dynamic suggests that supervision by ward sisters of their own staff might limit 'seeing beyond' the situation in terms of normal practice. Guided reflection can structure the clinical supervision. Johns and McCormack (Chapter 6) ask how a new technology like guided reflection can be implemented in meaningful and practical ways within everyday clinical practice. Guided reflection is an ideal technology, yet it is at risk of being accommodated within existing practice that threatens to nullify its therapeutic intention. It is easy to be sceptical that guided reflection will merely scratch the surface of practice when considering the minimal impact that other 'technologies', such as the nursing process, nursing models and named nursing, have generally had in changing practice. It must also be asked whether organisations want an empowered workforce. Indeed to suggest reflection as a process of empowerment suggests that nurses have to assert self against power gradients of more powerful others, whose own interests may be compromised. Nurses may have internalised a sense of the powerless self through working in bureaucratic settings which have taught everyone to be compliant, to be rule governed, and not to ask questions, seek alternatives or deal with competing values (Lieberman 1989). Smyth (1987) has noted:

> 'Most of us, unless we feel uncomfortable, shaken, or forced to look at ourselves and our circumstances, are unlikely to change. It is far easier to accept our current conditions and adopt the line of least resistance.' (p. 40)

These are important dynamics to understand because it cannot be expected that reflection can actually change practice when inserted into an unsympathetic culture. Indeed, guided reflection and clinical supervision will be accommodated to fit existing cultures. If this happens then its transformative potential will be nullified. Reflection will simply become technique focused. Van Manen (1977) identified three levels of reflection (Fig. 1.6). The technical and understanding levels accept the normative conditions of practice. Yet, it is only at the third 'conditions' level that cultural change can take place.

Technical level	Asking 'how' questions – how do I do something?
Understanding level	Asking 'why' questions – why should I respond in this way rather than that way? Why is this patient angry?
Conditions level	What are the underlying norms of practice that determine the way things are? Do these constrain desirable work? Can these be changed to facilitate desirable work?

Fig. 1.6   van Manen's three levels of reflection.

Illustrating the transformative potential

The impact of guided reflection is illustrated through Anäis's story (Chapter 7). The dialogue within guided reflection provides a rich sense and detail of the complexities, uncertainties and nuances of caring within everyday practice. Such dialogue can be analysed for an understanding of the meaning of practice and to see patterns through which transformation can be recognised. Factors that limit the transformative potential, either embodied within practitioners or embedded within the practice environment, can be identified and understood, and worked towards change.

This account gives meaning to Jean Watson's assertion (chapter 18) that guidance offers the practitioner a light, a way of seeing through the dark glass. Anäis is helped to see herself within the context of her practice. She can begin to make sense of who she is, her fears, hopes, her concerns, and to visualise new ways of adopting caring–healing ways. Reflection, like transformation, is a process over time, not confined to the guidance session. It is lived out within each caring moment. When Anäis meets with her supervisor next time, she could reflect on her triumph. She has fulfilled her caring potential and rejoices in the moment.

Researching self through reflection

Using reflection as a research method to research self was the focus of Judy Lumby's doctoral work [Chapter 8]. Judy Lumby is a clinical professor, sitting astride the academic and clinical worlds. She views reflection as a way for practitioners to 'validate' their paradoxical lives. By this she acknowledges the real world of practice that constrains nurses from being the people they might want to be. Transformation is always in the real world stuff – a tramp through the swamp of everyday practice. It is not some glowing, mystical light. And yet, as Jean Watson highlights through her concept of a 'clinical caritas' (chapter 18), it is a reaching out for the sacred within everyday practice, to realise what caring means even when the swamp seems all-consuming. Through her work with Maree and other practitioners, Judy Lumby paints a picture of a brave new world full of possibility for practitioners, researchers and educators. Her work opens doors to visualise a research tradition grounded in reflective practice. This builds on Bev Taylor's exploration of reflection as interpretative and critical phenomenology (Chapter 11).

We feel the reclaiming of story-telling is a most significant development. This confronts the reduction of story-telling to the status of anecdote that has no scientific credibility when viewed within the rules of what counts as valid evidence. Yet all nursing work is contextual. Nursing takes place within specific situations and always involves human encounter between two or more people. Such situations are never predictable, although how people respond in such situations is always informed by previous experience and knowledge. To argue otherwise, that such situations can be predictable, leads to a sterile world that reduces the practitioner to some kind of technician applying the rules, and the person being cared for to some object to be manipulated. This is so obvious, and yet why do nurses as researchers and educators continue to deny this fact? Why do they cling to out-moded illusions that limit rather than strengthen nursing's caring quest? The antidote can be glimpsed through Judy Lumby's work, where the uniqueness of person and situation is acknowledged as primary. Only in this way can transformation of self and situation be possible.

Reflection within practice

The focus of this discussion, and the early chapters of the book, illustrates and analyses the concept of reflection-on-experience. But who or what is a reflective practitioner? Is it someone who reflects-on-experience after the event, in her diary, within her clinical supervision, at home or on her educational course? Or is it someone who naturally sees and responds to each unfolding clinical moment through a reflective lens? I hope I have given a glimpse of reflection-in-action within Melissa's story. Without doubt, practitioners become increasingly sensitive to themselves within practice as a consequence of reflection-on-experience. Schön (1987) might describe this reflection as 'reflection-in-action'. He notes:

> 'We may reflect in the midst of action without interrupting it ... our thinking serves to reshape what we are doing while we are doing it.' (p. 26)

However, Schön discusses this concept as a response to a surprise within the smooth running of activity. I would argue that it is more than this, that it represents a deep sensitivity to even the smooth running of activity, a constant monitoring of self within the situation that ripples along the surface of conscious thought. It is better described as 'reflection-within-the moment' . Carolyn Moore and Julia Carter (Chapter 9) describe their action research project to implement reflection in practice. Julia's reflections illustrate that learning through reflection is essentially a subliminal learning through experience, recognised by looking back over time and seeing self as a changed person. It is this looking back to see self as a changed person that enables the reflexive nature of learning through reflection to be made manifest. Julia's reflective lens is structured through the reflective cues within the Burford NDU Model: Caring in Practice (Johns 1994b). Over time, Julia has internalised these cues as natural ways of seeing and responding to her clinical practice in ways that are congruent with her beliefs and values about her nursing practice. In this way these beliefs are realised as everyday practice.

The Burford NDU Model: Caring in Practice heralds a new generation of nursing models based on reflective and caring principles. The model justaposes and weaves nursing theory with reflective theory towards developing a reflective theory of nursing. This development is currently reflected in a set of explicit assumptions (Fig. 1.7).

- Caring in practice is grounded in a valid philosophy for practice underpinned by the unifying concept of human caring (Watson 1985).
- Inside every nurse there is a humanist struggling to get out, committed and active to realise caring in practice.
- All persons are seen and responded to as unitary human beings (Rogers 1986).
- The nurse works with the other through a continuing advocacy dialogue (Gadow 1980), mirrored by an internal dialogue with self (reflection-within-the moment).
- The intent of nursing is to enable the other towards realising recovery and growth as expanding consciousness (Newman 1994), through appropriate caring–healing responses.
- The extent to which the nurse can realise caring in practice is determined by the extent she is available to work with the person (Johns 1996).
- Growth is a mutual process of realisation.
- Caring in practice is manifest, known, and developed through reflection-on-experience.
- Caring in practice is a responsive and reflexive form in context with the environment in which it is practised.

Fig. 1.7 The Burford NDU Model: Caring in Practice explicit assumptions.

Julia's reflections illustrate the meaning of existential advocacy (Gadow 1980) as she strove to enable the patient to find meaning in their experience, and on this basis to make good decisions about their lives. Her reflections are part of a complementary dialogue with herself/her supervisor as she strove to find meaning in her practice. Each assumption of the model is as applicable to the practitioner as to the patient. 'Growth is a mutual process of realisation' applies to both the practioner and patient, and for the practitioner and her supervisor within guided reflection. In using a reflective model for nursing, the practitioner writes a reflective narrative of her unfolding experience with the patient. The nursing process is discarded because of its inappropriateness to the reflective practitioner. Writing a reflective narrative creates the opportunity for reflection as integral to everyday practice.

Another action research project to monitor the impact of introducing reflection-on-experience is described by Iain Graham (Chapter 10). Iain illustrates reflection as both a developmental process and as a collaborative way of structuring an action research process. He describes this process as 'phenomenological' reflection. The reader can appreciate the meaning of this within Bev Taylor's comparison of 'interpretative' and 'critical' reflection (Chapter 11).

Perhaps all reflection is phenomenological in the sense that it intends to find meaning within lived experience. The action research process takes this forward towards taking action based on these understandings within a continuous reflective spiral of action–reflection–action. The deconstruction of everyday lived experience creates a rich, contextual and subjective picture of the nuances of caring and the factors that influence this. At this level caring becomes visible. Becoming visible it becomes valued as making a difference in people's lives. Becoming valued, it is empowering.

Iain's account is infused with this notion of empowerment for the practitioners within the study as meaning unfolds and caring beliefs become realised in practice. It is the detailed study of transformation over time. Iain's work contributes to a guided reflection genre that offers a model for clinical practice and post-registration development. Bev Taylor frames reflection within a phenomenological research tradition as a link between an interpretative and critical paradigm. This fits in with certain theories of reflection (van Manen 1977; Mezirow 1981; Kemmis 1985) that help the practitioner to cross the critical threshold, as a way of understanding how the conditions under which practitioners practice can limit the achievement of desirable work. Through reflection the oppressive nature of these conditions can be understood towards establishing a critical and reflexive theory of practice.

Iain's research is complemented by Jane Glaze's research (Chapter 12). She utilises the work of Benner and Schön to demonstrate how she made these theories personally meaningful through the research process. Jane illustrates the impact of reflection to enable practitioners to understand and develop 'expert' practice with exemplars from her research respondents' practice.

These chapters have all been concerned with enabling practitioners to know and realise desirable work. It is easy to get tied up with the small issues of everyday practice from a reflective practice viewpoint. Indeed that has been the starting point of this book. Without knowing what is desirable, how can effective practice be known? Without a strong vision of what is desirable, transformation becomes a blurred horizon. The risk is that the practitioner will stumble in this haze of uncertainty, to sink in the swamplands of practice she inhabits. Tina Nordman and her colleagues (Chapter 13) explore reflection as a way of accessing the dialectic between hope and suffering within a broader canvas of human caring. It is significant to include contributions from different perspectives from across the world. Indeed there is a strong tradition of reflection and supervision in Scandinavia. Including this contribution firmly grounds transformation as human caring. It exemplifies nursing's quest to understand and assert human caring within everyday practice, and the realisation of nurses' therapeutic potential.

Reflection as knowing self

Reflection by its very nature is a very personal experience. The focus is on self in the context of self's practice. It exposes self to scrutiny. In this respect reflection may be disconcerting as taken for granted competence and ways of coping with anxiety are exposed as inadequate. Indeed, reflection may create crisis for practitioners as normal coping mechanisms are exposed as incongruent with achieving desirable work.

Exposing contradiction may increase frustration with work especially when new ways of responding to situations are not easily achieved. The fact that practitioners rationally know how they would like to respond in certain situations does not mean they can actually respond in these ways. Practice norms are deeply embodied and not so easily shrugged aside, especially when constructed and constantly reinforced by power relationships. Knowing self is pre-requisite to working with patients and families in helping them achieve their health needs (Johns 1996). In coming to know self, practitioners need to be aware of how their 'baggage' can interfere with seeing the concerns of the patient or the family (Hall 1964). Only by knowing her own baggage can the practitioner put it aside to be dealt with separately.

Dawn Freshwater (Chapter 14) constructs an analogy of alchemy to illustrate a reflective journey. Reflection is shown as a tool which allows the practitioner to penetrate the surface of self, to travel deep into the underworld of the subconscious. The alchemical process is discussed in three forms: the theoretical, the practical, and the transformative. The transformation takes place through a process of transmutation: after a difficult phase of angst (the blackening) comes a marriage of opposites, providing the opportunity for connection with the higher self. Dawn suggests that in order to 'transform lead into gold', we need to re-visit the 'prima materia' of everyday life. The challenge is for practitioners to revise the mundane through reflection and to review it as the sacred. Even within the 'blackness', practitioners can come to realise the joy that caring can be.

Stephen Wright (Chapter 15) picks up the theme of the sacred, reflection being a quest to reach and liberate the spiritual self. The notion of fulfilling the self's therapeutic potential is paralleled with fulfilling the self, to realise the self's human potential. Indeed, the two are the same thing. Reflection can create a clearing within the self, necessary in order to be open to the experience of others and to nurture the compassionate self.

The process of self becoming is further illustrated by Jan Bailey as she penetrates and learns through her own personal crisis (Chapter 16). Crisis is the moment of contradiction. Through reflection the crisis or contradiction is put into sharp focus. Practitioners tend to focus on experiences triggered by some emotional crisis. To reiterate, contradiction is the realisation that ways of living one's life are incongruous with one's beliefs. This is evident within many practitioners who say they value humanistic nursing and yet continue to practice in ways that reduce, that dishonours, the individual. Do they continue to lead false lives? Or can they confront the contradiction to resolve the contradiction, and in doing so honour themselves and those with whom they work?

Learning through crisis is transformation, moving from one level of functioning to a higher level.

This movement is central to Margaret Newman's theory of health as expanding consciousness (Newman 1994), in which the experience of suffering brings the practitioner into contact with the higher integrated self. This parallels the way the nurse works with the patient who presents in health crisis. From a caring reflective perspective, the practitioner establishes a caring dialogue to help the patient find meaning in the health event in order to make good decisions about their health/life. In doing so, old ways of living may be put into sharp context and become the focus for change. This is perhaps most evident where health events are life threatening, when the patient is confronted with the meaning of their life.

Margaret Newman draws on Arthur Young's theory of evolutionary consciousness to plot a journey of transformation through stages. The first stage is to understand events for what they are. The second stage is to see the choices a person has and to understand the consequences of those choices. The third stage is to 'unbind' self from behaving in certain ways that bind the person to normal ways of responding to situations. The fourth stage is empowerment, to take action based on new understandings and commitment to self. The fifth stage is transformation as the person steps out along this journey. The future cannot be predicted, although by being positive and true to self, it is a process of fulfilment and transformation. This is exactly the process of learning through reflection, and acknowledges the parallel process between therapeutic work within reflection and within clinical practice. The two are complementary. In freeing the self, the self is free to practise. Myra Davis (Chapter 17) continues this theme with her account of the way this inner struggle mirrors itself in the outer world of practice.

The wider perception

Finally, Jean Watson (Chapter 18) paints a contemporary post-modern landscape in which to view nursing's dilemma as to the tension within the nature of nursing's epistemological basis. She highlights the potentiality for reflective practice to find a way forward that honours both the visionary theorist philosopher, and honours the complexity of everyday practice. To reiterate, it is easy to get tied up with the small issues of everyday practice from a reflective practice viewpoint. Indeed, that is its starting point. Yet such work always needs to be informed by the practitioner's vision of what practice is about. Otherwise, how can a practitioner move towards desirable or effective practice, if what is desirable or what is effective practice is not known? Jean Watson offers an evolutionary perspective to consider this question. In doing so she posits reflective practice as an antithesis to theory driven practice, and begins to reorganise the arguments towards a juxtaposition where things are no longer divided, but simply in a dialectic tension. Vision is no elaborate fantasy, neither is it static. Through reflection the vision is constantly revisited and, as when moving across the landscape, the horizon is forever changing. To realise self is a process of transformation. It is forever.

Conclusion

Perhaps the answer to Jean's questions have to some extent been answered through the book. This is itself a moment for reflection as the reader gathers her thoughts. It is important to remember that this book, as a piece of reflective writing, does not set out to prescribe or predict the world. Theory and practice are not dichotomous. The illusion of separateness has served the needs of those who have made, and still make, such division. The illusion is that someone can enlighten, empower and transform another. Yet people can only enlighten, empower and transform themselves. But people can motivate, energise, inspire, challenge, support and inform others. Hopefully the reader will juxtapose the ideas within this book within her own reflective practice. The ideas within the book are simply another source of information to help the practitioner committed to creating a caring world, to achieve this through reflective practice.

References

Belenky, M.F., Clinchy, B.M., Goldberger, N.R. & Tarule, J.M. (1986) *Women's Ways of Knowing*. Basic Books, New York.

Benner, P. (1984) *From Novice to Expert*. Addison-Wesley, Menlo Park.

Boud, D., Keogh, R. & Walker, D. (1985) Promoting Reflection in Learning: a model. In *Reflection: Turning Experience into Learning*. (eds D. Boud, R. Keogh & D. Walker) p. 18–40. Kogan Page, London.

Boyd, E.M. & Fales, A.W. (1983) Reflective learning; key to learning from experience. *Journal of Humanistic Psychology*, **23**(2), 99–117.

Carper, B. (1978) Fundamental patterns of knowing in nursing. *Advances in Nursing Science*, **1**(1) 13–23.

Cox, H., Hickson, P. & Taylor, B. (1991) Exploring reflection: knowing and constructing practice. In *Toward a Discipline of Nursing* (eds R. Gray & R. Pratt). Churchill Livingstone, Melbourne.

Elcock, K. (1997) Reflections on being therapeutic and reflection. *Nursing in Critical Care*, **2**(3), 138–43.

Gadow, S. (1980) Existential Advocacy. In *Nursing: Image and Ideals* (eds S.F. Spicker & S. Gadow). Springer Publishing, New York.

Greenwood, J. (1993) Some considerations concerning practice and feedback in nursing education. *Journal of Advanced Nursing*, 18, 1999–2002.

Hall, L. (1964) Nursing – what is it? *The Canadian Nurse*, **60**(2), 150–54.

Johns, C. (1994a) Guided reflection. In *Reflective Practice in Nursing; the Growth of the Professional Practitioner* (eds A. Palmer, S. Burns & C. Bulman). Blackwell Science, Oxford.

Johns, C. (ed.) (1994b) *The Burford NDU Model: Caring in Practice.* Blackwell Science, Oxford.

Johns, C. (1995) Framing learning through reflection within Carper's fundamental ways of knowing. *Journal of Advanced Nursing,* 22, 226–34.

Johns, C. (1996) Visualising and realising caring in practice through guided reflection. *Journal of Advanced Nursing,* 24, 1135–43.

Johns, C. (1997a) Commentary on reflection – 'reflections on reflection'. *Nursing in Critical Care* **2**(3), 144–5.

Johns, C. (1997b) Commentary on reflection – 'reasonable refusal? an ethical dilemma'. *Nursing in Critical Care,* **2**(2), 81–2.

Johns, C. (1997c) *Becoming a reflective practitioner.* PhD thesis. The Open University, Milton Keynes.

Kelley, P. & Callanan, M. (1992) *Final Gifts: Understanding the Special Awareness, Needs and Communications of the Dying.* Bantam Books, New York.

Kemmis, S. (1985) Action research and the politics of reflection. In (eds D. Boud, R. Keogh & D. Walker) p. 139–64. Kogan Page, London.

Lieberman, A. (1989) *Staff Development in Culture Building, Curriculum and Teaching: the Next 50 Years.* Teachers' College Press, New York.

Mezirow, J. (1981) A critical theory of adult learning and education. *Adult Education,* **32**(1), 3–24.

Mishler, E. G. (1986) The analysis of interview – narratives. In Sarbin T.R. [ed.] *Narrative Psychology: The Storied Nature of Human Conduct* (ed. T.R. Sarbin) p. 111–25. Praeger, New York.

Newman, M. (1994) *Health as Expanding Consciousness,* 2nd edn. NLN, New York.

Newell, R. (1992) Anxiety, accuracy and reflection: the limits of professional development. *Journal of Advanced Nursing,* 17, 1326–33.

Reece Jones, P. (1995) Hindsight bias in reflective practice: an empirical investigation. *Journal of Advanced Nursing,* 21, 781–8.

Rogers, M. (1986) Science of unitary human beings. In *Explorations of Martha Rogers' Science of Unitary Human Beings* (ed. V. Malinkski), pp. 4–23. Appleton-Century-Crofts, Norwalk, CT.

Schön, D. A. (1983) *The Reflective Practitioner.* Avebury, Aldershot.

Schön, D.A. (1987) *Educating the Reflective Practitioner.* Jossey-Bass, San Francisco.

Smyth, J. (1987) *A Rationale for Teachers' Critical Pedagogy: A Handbook.* Deakin University Press, Victoria.

Strauss, A. & Corbin, J. (1990) *Basics of Qualitative Research.* Sage, Newberry Park.

Street, A. F. (1992) *Inside Nursing: A Critical Ethnography of Clinical Nursing.* SUNY, New York.

Van Manen, M. (1977) Linking ways of knowing with ways of being. *Curriculum Inquiry,* 6(3), 205–28.

Visinstainer, M.A. (1986) The nature of knowledge and theory in nursing. *Image: The Journal of Nursing Scholarship,* **18**, 32–8.

Watson, J. (1985) *Nursing: Human Science and Human Care: A Theory of Nursing.* National League for Nursing, New York.

White, J. (1995) Patterns of knowing: review, critique, and update. *Advances in Nursing Science,* **17**(4), 73–86.

Chapter 2
Beyond Expertise: Reflective and Reflexive Nursing Practice

Gary Rolfe

Introduction

Much has been written over the past decade about reflective practice in nursing, usually focusing on the benefits of reflection, or on procedural models and structures for engaging in it. This chapter seeks to explore two issues which the nursing literature has failed to address in any depth. Firstly, almost all the nurses writing about reflective practice have focused on what Schön (1983) referred to as reflection-*on*-action, that is, on retrospective reflection carried out after and usually away from the event. Schön's other form of reflection, reflection-*in*-action, which he also referred to as 'experimenting in action' or 'thinking on your feet', is hardly considered at all.

Secondly, although a great deal has been written about the 'mechanics' of reflective practice, most writers have kept silent about the underlying processes, or have avoided a detailed consideration by claiming that the practice of nursing is an intuitive art which defies conscious deliberation. However, as Schön (1983) pointed out:

> 'When people use terms such as "art" and "intuition", they usually intend to terminate discussion rather than to open up inquiry. It is as though the practitioner says to his academic colleague, "While I do not accept *your* view of knowledge, I cannot describe my own." Sometimes, indeed, the practitioner appears to say, "My kind of knowledge is indescribable," or even, "I will not attempt to describe it lest I paralyse myself." These attitudes have contributed to a widening rift between the universities and the professions, research and practice, thought and action.'

This chapter seeks to address both of the above issues by describing and discussing a reflexive approach to practice in which clinical judgements are formulated and tested in a conscious and mindful way.

Expertise and reflection-on-action

One of the contributing factors to the rise in popularity of reflective practice in nursing over the past 10 years must surely be Patricia Benner's influential book *From Novice to Expert* (Benner 1984). Benner suggested five levels of practice, from the rule-bound novice or beginner who nurses literally 'by the book', following non-contextualised rule-governed procedures, to the expert who:

> 'with an enormous background of experience, now has an intuitive grasp of each situation and zeroes in on the accurate region of the problem without wasteful consideration of a large range of unfruitful, alternative diagnoses and solutions.' (Benner 1984)

Benner based her notion of expertise on the work of brothers Hubert and Stuart Dreyfus, a philosopher and a computer scientist. The Dreyfus brothers were working in the field of artificial intelligence, and came to the conclusion that human experts process information entirely differently from computers. They used the example of a chess grandmaster to illustrate how the expert 'zeroes in' on a chess problem, arguing that unlike the computer, the grandmaster does not consider every possible move (clearly an impossible task), but draws on his or her experiential repertoire of similar board positions from past games. In the same way, claimed Benner, the expert nurse calls on a body of experiential knowledge – what she referred to as a repertoire of paradigm cases – and instinctively and intuitively matches the current situation with a paradigm case which has proved effective in a similar situation in the past.

Expertise is therefore an unconscious, intuitive process, which Benner, drawing on the terminology of the philosopher Gilbert Ryle (1963), referred to as 'know-how'. She claimed that this know-how consisted of tacit knowledge that did not follow a logical analytic process and could not be expressed in words, but is rather 'understanding without a rationale' (Benner & Tanner 1987). Furthermore, if the expert nurse does attempt to consciously gain access to her know-how, it mysteriously evaporates, such that 'if experts are made to attend to the particulars or to a formal model or rule, their performance actually deteriorates' (Benner 1984). The expert cannot say how she knows what to do, and if she deliberately tries to practise according to a conscious logical procedure, she is no longer functioning as an expert.

This can be seen clearly from examples such as driving a car or playing the piano. Expert car drivers or pianists are not conscious of their performance; they drive or play without having to pay attention to what they are doing. Expert drivers change up and down through the gears intuitively, and it is only when they are forced to consciously think about what they are doing that they make mistakes, as for example when driving a car they are not used to.

However, although the 'intuitive grasp' underpinning expert practice is unknown, and according to Benner, unknowable, it is not a magical process and 'intuitive grasp should not be confused with mysticism since it is available only in situations where a deep background understanding of the situation exists' (Benner 1984). Intuition is based on an experiential knowledge-base, on knowledge gleaned from individual concrete experiences, but Benner is quick to recognise that this experiential knowledge does not necessarily come merely from exposure to situations; not every nurse who has been practising for 20 years is an expert. Thus, 'experience, as the word is used here, does not refer to mere passage of time or longevity', and 'there is a leap, a discontinuity, between the competent level and the proficient and expert levels' (Benner 1984). Clearly, something has to be done with the experience to transform it into expertise; it needs to be processed. Benner had probably not read the work of Donald Schön when she was writing her book (Schön's seminal work *The Reflective Practitioner* was published only a year before Benner's), but if she had, she would surely have recognised the process of turning experience into the knowledge-base of expertise as what Schön (1983) referred to as reflection-on-action.

For Schön, reflection-on-action was a way of generating knowledge from the messy and unpredictable 'swampy lowland' of the practice setting, by actively processing experiences after, and usually away from, the situation in which those experiences were acquired. Reflection-on-action can therefore be summarised as:

> 'the retrospective contemplation of practice undertaken in order to uncover the knowledge used in a particular situation, by analyzing and interpreting the information recalled. The reflective practitioner may speculate how the situation might have been handled differently and what other knowledge would have been helpful.' (Fitzgerald 1994)

Two necessary conditions for reflection-on-action are highlighted in this definition. Firstly, as Andrews (1996) pointed out, the experience must be actively processed if it is to be converted into knowledge, and 'reflection is, therefore, not to be confused with thinking about practice, which may only involve recalling what has occurred rather than learning from it'. And secondly, reflection-on-action can only take place after the event. It is *retrospective* contemplation of practice, and as Van Manen (1990) noted:

> 'a person cannot reflect on lived experience while living through the experience. For example, if one tries to reflect on one's anger while being angry, one finds that the anger has already changed or dissipated. Thus, phenomenological reflection is not *introspective* but *retrospective*. Reflection on lived experience is always recollective; it is reflection on experience that is already passed or lived through.'

This is an important point; if we attempt to reflect on an experience while we are still immersed in it, then the reflection on that experience changes the nature of the experience itself. Schön (1983) referred to this kind of reflection as reflection-*in*-action, and as we have seen, reflection-in-action is not only reflective but reflexive, changing the nature of the situation while we are in it.

To take Van Manen's example: by reflecting *on* our anger, after and away from the situation in which it occurred, we can learn some important lessons about the nature of that anger and its effect on ourselves and others, and this learning can contribute to our repertoire of paradigm cases. But by reflecting *during* our anger, we transform it into something else. We are no longer angry, or at least, our anger has to some extent dissipated. Furthermore, by reflecting on our new mental state, that too is transformed; we are not only generating knowledge about the situation we find ourselves in, but in the process of generating knowledge we are changing the situation in a reflexive spiral.

It could reasonably be argued, then, that although Benner was probably not aware of Schön's work while she was writing her book *From Notice to Expert*, the process which Schön described as reflection-on-action is very similar to the way in which Benner envisaged the expert nurse as processing her experiences and turning them into paradigm cases. What Benner's expert was *not* doing was reflection-in-action, what Schön (1983) called 'thinking on your feet', which requires a conscious attention to the underlying thought processes of practice actually during that practice. This can be seen quite clearly in Benner's account of an expert psychiatric nurse attempting to explain her clinical judgement:

> 'When I say to a doctor "the patient is psychotic", I don't always know how to legitimize the statement. But I am never wrong, because I know psychosis from inside out. And I feel that, and I know it, and I trust it.' (Benner 1984)

As the nurse says, she cannot legitimize her statement with a reasoned chain of argument; she simply *feels* that she is right (and, as Benner pointed out, she probably is!).

As we have noted, Benner was heavily influenced by the work of Drefus and Dreyfus on expert computer systems, and it was these writers who introduced her to the idea that human experts employ an unconscious pattern-matching strategy in their practice. Dreyfus and Dreyfus (1986) cited an experiment in which a chess grandmaster carried out complex mental arithmetic whilst playing chess, and noted that his game was hardly affected. This led them to the conclusion that intuitive grasp transcended logical thought, and accounts for the fact that Benner's expert psychiatric nurse could make complex clinical decisions without understanding the rationale behind them. There simply was no rationale. The nurse could be mentally compiling a shopping list (or, indeed, doing mental arithmetic), and her judgement would be unaffected.

For Benner's expert, then, the conscious, rational thought processes take place after and away from practice; it is through reflection-on-action that raw experience is transformed into paradigm cases, which are then somehow matched to whatever clinical situation the nurse might find herself in. And if she has no cases which match the situation, then she has to return to a lower level of practice and consciously think out her next move, but this of course results in inferior judgements.

The limitations of expertise

Although now widely accepted by the nursing profession, this model of expertise is not without its critics. The most common objection is that Benner's model of expertise as unknowable intuitive grasp leads to a form of elitism in which self-styled experts need not justify their practice to the 'lower orders' of nurses. Like Benner's psychiatric nurse, the expert is never wrong, and because her expertise is unfathomable, it is also safe from attack; she does not have to justify her decisions because she *cannot* justify her decisions. She just knows that she is always right.

There is, however, a more important and far-reaching objection to Benner's notion of the intuitive expert. Whilst unconscious intuitive grasp, whether it is employed in diagnosing psychosis or in driving a car, might lead to smooth, effortless, spontaneous practice in which conscious thought is not required, it also has certain dangers:

> 'As a practice becomes more repetitive and routine, and as knowing-in-practice becomes increasingly tacit and spontaneous, the practitioner may miss important opportunities to think about what he is doing. He may find that . . . he is drawn into patterns of error which he cannot correct. And if he learns, as often happens, to be selectively inattentive to phenomena that do not fit the categories of his knowing-in-action, then he may suffer from boredom or "burn out" and afflict his clients with the consequences of his narrowness and rigidity. When this happens, the practitioner has "over-learned" what he knows.' (Schön 1983)

The expert might well be able to nurse and do mental arithmetic at the same time, but if she does, then an important learning experience will be lost to her. And furthermore, by restricting her reflective practice to reflection-*on*-action, to what Van Manen earlier referred to as retrospection rather than introspection, she is leaving the development of her practice largely to chance, to the unknown and unknowable process of intuitive grasp and pattern matching.

When most nurses write about reflective practice they are referring almost exclusively to reflection-on-action, the retrospective contemplation of practice, and when reflection-in-action is mentioned, it is usually rather obliquely. Detailed explorations of reflection-in-action are unusual in the nursing journals, partly because this conflicts with Benner's notion of expertise, and because as we have seen, 'if experts are made to attend to the particulars . . . their performance actually deteriorates'. (Benner 1984)

The legacy of Benner's model is therefore almost a denial that reflection-in-action is possible. As Dreyfus and Dreyfus (1986) pointed out:

> 'Have you ever been driving effortlessly along a city street in a stick-shift car and suddenly found yourself consciously thinking about the gear you are in and whether it's appropriate? Chances are the sudden reflection upon what you were doing [reflection-in-action] and the rules for doing it was accompanied by a severe degradation of performance; perhaps you shifted at the wrong time or into the wrong gear.'

Dreyfus and Dreyfus are undoubtedly correct in their observation that reflection-in-action detracts from driving a car, but the flaw in their argument is to attempt to apply the same model to cognitive decision-making processes such as chess playing or clinical nursing judgements. Motor skills such as driving a car rely on an interplay between brain, body and eye which circumvents rational cognition, and as most expert car drivers and pianists will tell you, their performance does indeed degenerate when attended to.

However, cognitive abilities such as chess playing and making clinical judgements are of a different order, and whereas expertise in motor skills is acquired by repeated mechanical practice, the expertise of a chess grandmaster is clearly not. As Dreyfus and Dreyfus (1986) themselves pointed out:

> 'Not all people achieve expert levels in their skills. Some areas of skill – chess, for example – have the characteristics that only a very small fraction of beginners can ever master the domain ... Other areas, such as automobile driving, are so designed that almost all novices can eventually reach the level we call expert.'

The difference between chess and driving is not merely a difference of degree as Dreyfus and Dreyfus seem to be suggesting; it is the difference between a motor skill and an advanced and complex cognitive ability. For the vast majority of people, no amount of practice will ever result in their becoming a chess grandmaster because expertise in chess is not acquired in the same way as expertise in driving, but requires an active, conscious process of introspection.

Thus, while unconscious expertise is the highest stage of attainment for motor skills, cognitive abilities are somewhat different. Dreyfus and Dreyfus (1986) themselves recognised this when they asked the question: 'What does a masterful chess player think about when time permits, even when an intuitively obvious move has come spontaneously to mind?'

The answer, they tell us, is that he or she thinks about chess in a process of 'deliberative rationality', unlike the expert car driver who generally thinks about anything but driving. Of course, the chess grandmaster does not *have* to think about chess. They can, as Dreyfus and Dreyfus demonstrated, do mental arithmetic, and their performance will not be significantly impaired. But the point is that thinking about chess will make a better chess player in a way that thinking about driving will not make for a better driver. As Van Manen pointed out, reflection-in-action changes the situation in which the reflection is taking place, but unlike with motor skills, when we are reflecting about cognitive process the changes are not necessarily for the worse.

Beyond expertise

A number of writers are now coming to recognise the limitations of Benner's model, and are arguing that although what she called 'intuitive grasp' might well be unconscious, it is not unknowable. Brook and Champion (1991) rejected the notion of irrational intuition and argued that expert performance involves the formulation and testing of hypotheses during the process of practice. Elstein & Bordage (1988) pointed out that 'it seems practically impossible to reason without hypotheses whenever the data base is as complex as it typically is in clinical problems', and Andrews (1996) claimed that so-called intuition is a complex critical skill closely related to reflection-in-action. And as Schön (1987) noted:

> 'When the practitioner reflects in action in a case he perceives as unique, paying attention to phenomena and surfacing his intuitive understanding of them, his experience is at once exploratory, move testing, and hypothesis testing. The three functions are fulfilled by the very same actions. And from this fact follows the distinctive character of experimenting in practice.' (Schön 1987)

It would appear then that intuition might not be the unknowable and irrational process that Benner made it out to be, but rather an unconscious form of hypothesis construction and testing. Even Benner herself appeared to recognise this when she wrote that 'expertise develops when the clinician tests and refines propositions, hypotheses, and principle-based expectations in actual practice situations' (Benner 1984). And if the process is rational and knowable, then it should be possible to elevate it into consciousness. Indeed, there is evidence to suggest that some nurses actually *do* make clinical decisions by employing a conscious process of hypothesising (Skinner & Rolfe 1996).

It might on first sight seem that the only difference between conscious and unconscious hypothesising is simply that one is a conscious process whilst the other is not. However, as Van Manen pointed out earlier, conscious reflection-in-action entails a reflexivity which modifies the object of the reflection and has a direct impact on the practice situation. Expertise and reflection-in-action might look the same, but whereas the expert is acting intuitively and without conscious thought, almost at spinal cord level, reflection-in-action requires a particular sort of mindfulness which involves intense concentration on the task at hand, and has a direct impact on the situation in which it is taking place. Thus:

> 'When someone reflects-in-action, he becomes a researcher in the practice context. He is not dependent on the categories of established theory and technique, but constructs a new theory of the unique case ... because his experimenting is a kind of action, implementation is built into his inquiry.' (Schön 1983)

Practice based on conscious reflection-in-action therefore moves beyond expertise. Whereas the expert is a reflective practitioner who builds up a repertoire of paradigm cases through reflection-on-action, which she then applies through unconscious pattern matching, the nurse who is employing conscious reflection-in-action is a reflexive practitioner who directly modifies her practice on the spot in response to her hypothesis testing. Even with very simple and seemingly mechanical tasks such as wound dressing, the difference is striking: the expert nurse would perform the required actions swiftly and deftly and without conscious thought, whereas the reflexive practioner would think about every move, every decision, relating them to this patient in this situation.

More importantly, the reflexive practitioner would be learning from her performance, thinking about how it could be done differently, constructing theories, testing hypotheses, and modifying her actions on the spot, and this requires mindful attention. Reflection-in-action therefore serves to focus the concentration of the reflexive practitioner on the here-and-now and on the uniqueness of her individual relationship with each of her patients, and reduces the possibility of boredom and burn out that comes from overfamiliarity with the tasks to be performed.

In fact, the notion of reflexive practice, in which hypotheses are formulated and tested in a continuous spiral, is not a new idea in nursing, and is implicit in the nursing process cycle of assessment, planning, implementing the plan and evaluating the outcome, which in turn leads to a new assessment of the transformed situation. The process is also recognised in education and research. Kolb's learning cycle (Kolb 1975) contains the elements of observation and reflection on an experience, conceptualizing an explanation for that experience, active experimentation based on the explanation, and new reflections on the transformed situation. Similarly, the action research spiral includes 'repeated cycles of analysis, reconnaissance, problem reconceptualisation, planning, implementation of social action, and evaluation' (McKernan 1991).

The central feature of all these models is the notion of constructing a personal theory based on an individual assessment of the situation, the testing of that theory in a real life setting, and the subsequent modification of the theory. In each case, the model is self-reflexive; it both modifies the practice situation and is itself modified by the changes it brings about. Thus, the reflexive practitioner is not only learning from a situation by formulating personal theories which express her understanding of it, but she is also changing the situation by testing out hypotheses derived from those theories in the clinical situation.

The fact that this process involves hypothesis generation and testing should not lead us to associate it with the hypothetico-deductivism of the scientific method. The hypotheses or theories that the reflexive practitioner forms are theories which account for a specific situation, and are not intended to be generalized beyond that situation. Furthermore, they are a synthesis of scientific knowledge from empirical research, experiential knowledge drawn from similar clinical encounters, and personal knowledge about herself and this particular patient. Reflexive practice consists not only of the possession of these very different forms of knowledge, but in knowing how to combine them to form the most likely hypothesis or personal theory: how much weight to give each element, which to include and which to leave out, and how to choose between competing hypotheses.

I believe that there is a logic to this process of clinical judgement, but that it is not the formal logic of science. Rather, I have suggested elsewhere (Rolfe 1996) that the expert nurse employs a form of induction known as abductivism (Pierce 1958) which turns formal Aristotelian logic on its head. In claiming that expertise is rational, I am therefore not suggesting that it follows the logic of empirical science, merely that it is a logical and potentially understandable process. This, of course, is in direct contrast to Benner's position that expertise is unknown and unknowable and that it is a form of intuition.

It is not my contention that intuition does not exist, nor that nurses do not sometimes rely on it in their practice, merely that Benner has fallen into the logical trap of the principle of the excluded middle: that expertise is either based on scientific logic or else it is based on no logic at all. Contrary to what many scientists would have us believe, there are other logics and other rationalities besides those of the scientific method, and rather than expending time and energy saying what expertise is not, perhaps we should be actively exploring what it is.

Conclusion

I have argued in this chapter that whereas Benner's fifth and final level of expert might be appropriate for activities based largely on motor skills, professions which rely on advanced cognitive abilities such as on-the-spot decision making and clinical judgement will benefit from a conscious, reflexive level of practice which goes beyond expertise. The reflexive practitioner, unlike Benner's expert, is consciously shaping and modifying her practice through a process of theorising and hypothesis testing in direct response to feedback from, and evaluation of, her previous actions. She is therefore constantly learning from her practice by developing theories which attempt to explain it, and she checks out her learning by testing the theories in her own practice.

But the reflexive practitioner is not only *acquiring* knowledge; she is also *generating* it through on-the-spot experimenting in a process which looks a lot like the action research cycle of 'a circle of planning, action, and fact-finding about the result of the action' (Lewin 1946). Thus, by reflecting-in-action, the nurse integrates education and research into her everyday practice.

This model of the practitioner as an active learner and researcher challenges many of the nursing profession's existing notions about education and research. It implies a revision in the current educational philosophy inherent in Project 2000 nurse training, of a technocratic model in which theory is taught in universities and colleges of higher education and is then expected to be applied to practice situations (Bines 1992). It also challenges the Department of Health's elitist strategy for research in which 'not ... all practitioners should be carrying out research as part of their professional role or professional development' (DoH 1993).

Most importantly, however, the reflexive practitioner, unlike the expert, is able to justify her clinical decisions and provide reasoned argument for acting the way she did. This is of particular significance given the Department of Health's current drive towards 'evidence-based practice', and whereas the expert cannot always justify her statements (she just *knows* that she is always right!), the reflexive practitioner can produce evidence for her actions, albeit not necessarily the kind of evidence that the DoH had in mind.

But if nursing is to move forward as a profession, then we must not only do, but be able to describe what we do and how we do it. The expert's defence that her practice is unknowable is not good enough; we must uncover the rational process behind our decisions and judgements (even though it might not be the rationality of western empirical science), and reflection-in-action is one much overlooked way of doing so.

References

Andrews, M. (1996) Using reflection to develop clinical expertise. *British Journal of Nursing*, **5**(8), 508–13.

Benner, P. (1984) *From Novice to Expert*. Addison-Wesley, Menlo Park.

Benner, P. & Tanner, C. (1987) Clinical judgement: how expert nurses use intuition. *American Journal of Nursing*, **87** (1), 23–31.

Bines, H. (1992) Issues in course design. In *Developing Professional Education* (eds H. Bines & D. Watson). Open University Press, Buckingham.

Brook, V. & Champion, E. (1991) *The Reflective Practitioner*. Fairway Publications, Tiverton.

DoH (1993) *Report of the Taskforce on the Strategy for Research in Nursing, Midwifery and Health Visiting*. HMSO, London.

Dreyfus, H.L. & Dreyfus, S.E. (1986) *Mind Over Machine*. Basil Blackwell, Oxford.

Elstein, A.S. & Bordage, G. (1988) Psychology of clinical reasoning. In *Professional Judgement* (eds J. Downie & A. Elstein). Cambridge University Press, Cambridge.

Fitzgerald, M. (1994) Theories of reflection for learning. In *Reflective Practice in Nursing* (eds A. Palmer, S. Burns & C. Bulman) Blackwell Science, Oxford.

Kolb, D.A. & Fry, R. (1975) Towards an applied theory of experiential learning. In *The Theories of Group Processes* (ed. D. Cooper). John Lilley & Sons, London.

Lewin, K. (1946) Action research and minority problems. *Journal of Social Issues*, **2**, 34–46.

McKernan, J. (1991) *Curriculum Action Research*. Kogan Page, London.

Peirce, C.S. (1958) *Collected Papers*j vol. VII. Harvard University Press, Cambridge, MA.

Rolfe, G. (1996) *Closing the Theory–Practice Gap*. Butterworth Heinemann, Oxford.

Ryle, G. (1963) *The Concept of Mind*. Penguin, Harmondsworth.

Schön, D.A. (1983) *The Reflective Practitioner*. Temple Smith, London.

Schön, D.A. (1983) *The Reflective Practitioner*. Temple Smith, London.

Schön, D.A. (1987) *Educating the Reflective Practitioner*. Jossey-Bass, San Francisco.

Skinner, M. & Rolfe, G. (1996) The role of hypothesising and intuition in advanced practice. In *Closing the Theory-Practice Gap* (G. Rolfe). Butterworth Heinemann, Oxford.

Van Manen, M. (1990) *Researching Lived Experience*. State University of New York Press, New York.

Chapter 3

Doing the Right Thing: Customary vs Reflective Morality in Nursing Practice

Lucie Ferrell

Introduction

Resolving moral issues and dilemmas in nursing practice has long been an area of professional concern. Historically, the traditional ethic has been the perspective that doing the right thing can be determined by previous decisions or following traditional norms of nursing, or by an appeal to an ethic of pure altruism, thus demonstrating a customary morality as standard practice. However, given the current health care environment of economic constraints, legal accountability, personal–professional conflicts, and moral complexities, this approach is deemed too simplistic to be useful or to offer resolution to moral issues. Ethical practice of nursing demands a reflective morality, dictating a thoughtful analysis of moral issues and dilemmas as well as a consideration of the person who is nurse, her values, beliefs, and the meaning she attributes to being a nurse. This reflective morality require the nurse to relinquish the comfort of 'following orders' and the traditional 'way we've always done it' and to adopt the personal and professional standard of moral autonomy. It is through this reflective morality that the nurse is empowered to do the right thing in her practice of nursing.

In developing this thesis, the nurse is viewed as a moral agent whose endeavours are designed to bring about good and whose practice occurs in the moral universe that is health care. The nurse is also, therefore, in a position to cause harm to patients through her actions, both directly and indirectly. Further, the nurse is an autonomous professional and a licensed practitioner, both of which carry legal implications, and she is most often an employee of a health care institution with accompanying moral obligations and constraints. As a basic consideration, however, this nurse is a person. This person who is a nurse has values and beliefs, life goals, other social roles and obligations, life experiences and personal moral rights; all of these are factors to consider in a discussion of transforming practice through reflective morality. These are identified as the dimensions of professional nursing practice: the ethical, the socio-legal, the legal-regulatory, the economic, and the personal dimensions and comprise a framework for reflection and analysis when confronting moral issues and dilemmas in nursing practice (Ferrell 1992).

The nurse as moral agent

Professional practice standards require that the nurse act in accordance with ethical principles and in a manner that does not harm patients entrusted to her care. The profession of nursing exists to provide care to patients and it is excellent care that is the 'primary moral imperative' of nursing practice (Bishop & Scudder 1990, p. 113); good, defined as patient health and wellbeing, is the goal of that care. Because nursing actions are designed to bring about good for the patient, it follows that the nurse, through her actions, has the capability of harming the patient as well, either directly or indirectly, knowingly or unintentionally.

This potential for causing harm demands that the nurse be ethical in her practice of nursing, that her nursing judgements, decisions and actions be sound and morally right. Because of this inherent capacity for causing harm as well as good, the health care environment is viewed as a moral universe, and nursing, as a health care profession, is a moral endeavour (Bandman & Bandman 1990; Jameton 1984; Bishop & Scudder 1990). In this sense of nursing as a moral endeavour, the nurse is a moral agent responsible and accountable for her practice: her judgements, her actions, and the consequences of these. Every professional judgement and nursing action has an ethical dimension because each of these, directly or indirectly, affects the wellbeing of patients.

> 'More than any other discipline, the practitioner of nursing is in continuous contact with the patient and the family. This position offers unique privileges and responsibilities.' (Bandman and Bandman 1990, p. 2)

Relative to moral agency, Engelhardt (1986) identifies nurses as 'in-between' in that nurses are caught 'in-between' the traditional authority of the physician, the emerging concept of patient rights, and the growing power of hospital bureaucrats. Placement among these various factions makes it difficult for nurses to make ethical decisions. Yarling and McElmurry (1986) develop this idea of the 'in-between' position of the nurse and argue that nurses are not free to act as they feel morally compelled to act. The authors maintain that:

> 'the fundamental moral predicament of hospital nurses is that they often are not free to be moral because they often are not free, due to institutional constraints, to exercise their commitment to the patient through excellence in patient care.' (p. 130)

It is their contention that nurses lack sufficient autonomy to be moral agents because of such institutional constraints.

Bishop and Scudder, in their landmark text *The Practical, Moral, and*

Personal Sense of Nursing (1990), refute this stance with philosophical argument stating that:

> 'The in-between place of the nurse does not free her from the responsibility of making moral decisions; instead, it sets the context in which these decisions must be made.' (p. 137)

Further, they maintain that excellent practice is the primary moral imperative for nurses and that conflict over competing rights obscures the moral agency of the patient and the nurse. They discuss the inherent moral dilemmas in nursing practice and differentiate between the medically right decision, as decided by the physician, and the morally good decision, as decided by the patient (p. 116).

The moral agency of the nurse is consistent with the statement by Taylor (1975):

> 'A moral agent is any being who is capable of thinking, deciding, and acting in accordance with moral standards and rules. A moral agent may not always fulfill the requirements of a moral standard or rule; that is, he need not be morally perfect. But he must have the capacity to judge himself on the basis of such a criterion and to use it as a guide to his choice and conduct.' (p. 6)

The implications for a requirement of reflection on the part of a moral agent are clear in this definition and it is this that determines the moral agency of the nurse. In the current consideration, the nurse is viewed as a moral agent in that she possesses individual ability to affect the good of the patient as well as to cause harm and she holds moral accountability for her practice. She is capable of thinking, deciding and acting in accordance with moral standards and rules. What is more, as a health care professional, she is expected to do so.

As an autonomous professional, the nurse is held legally accountable for her practice. There is a public trust which mandates that the professional must act in accord with the best interests of patients, will not cause them harm, and will hold herself accountable for professional nursing care. This social contract of trust between the professions and society defines the legal contract in terms of the nurse-patient relationship. The nurse is held legally accountable for her actions as a trusted professional and, should she violate that trust, will be subject to legal sanctions. Likewise, as a licensed practitioner, the nurse is subject to legal-regulatory standards and is held accountable for meeting these. Should she fail to do so, again the nurse will experience legal consequences. These legal accountabilities, as well as the moral accountability, contribute to the complexity of moral dilemmas and issues in nursing practice and so must be considered in a reflective morality.

Adding to this complexity is the fact that most nurses are employees of bureaucratic institutions, inherently a situation of conflict because, as a professional, the nurse is autonomous – accountable to ethical and professional standards – yet, as an employee, she experiences employer control and is subject to employer standards and constraints. Further, within a hospital which, because its business is health care, has moral obligations to society and to the patient, there are rules designed to assist the hospital in meeting these moral obligations. Such rules carry with them the weight of the moral imperative and, therefore, employees have the moral obligation to follow them (Purtilo & Cassel 1981). A professional has been described as one who is bound by values and standards other than those of his or her employing organisation, and hence the built-in potential for conflict. Again, this is a factor which greatly increases the complexity of ethical decision-making.

As a healthcare provider, the nurse must practise with moral integrity and professional commitment, maintaining and safeguarding her patients' wellbeing as well as that of her own., She is expected to act 'with courage' when confronting injustice (Purtilo & Cassel, 1981, p. 35); with integrity where encountering potential harm to patients; with compassion in her daily work of nursing; with a constant willingness to place patient welfare as her highest priority; and with excellent practice as her moral obligation. The 'art of care' and the 'moral sense' (Bishop & Scudder 1990) join, not only in the professional relationship that is nursing, but also within the person who is nurse. This personal dimension is a critical dimension because it is the person who is nurse who brings to her practice the life experiences, personal values and beliefs, life goals and meaning, and who must incorporate these into a reflective morality if she is to uphold the professional standard of moral autonomy. It is this standard which provides the impetus for moving from a customary morality to a reflective morality, the hallmark of professional practice.

Customary vs reflective morality

'The ultimate purpose of normative and analytic ethics is to enable us to arrive at a critical reflective morality of our own' (Taylor 1975, p. 9). This is especially true for the person who is nurse, one who bears moral accountability for her practice and who is the practitioner of the moral art of nursing. As a moral agent, the nurse in her daily practice is concerned with ethical issues, making decisions that will be judged as right or wrong, affecting the wellbeing of those patients in her care. In this sense, it is critical how the nurse actualises the moral practice of nursing. Taylor (1975) defines moral maturity as:

'the condition in which an individual has the capacity to be open-minded about his moral beliefs, defending them by reasoned argument when they are challenged and giving them up when they are shown to be false or unjustified.' (p. 10)

Individuals are reared with some set of moral beliefs and in a society with some kind of moral code that is its norm. The person may either blindly accept this moral code, thus operating from a customary morality, or may reflect upon it, critically analyse it, and then adopt or reject it, in part or in whole, as her own moral code. Moral growth occurs as the person develops the capacity to reason about her moral values and beliefs. She thinks clearly, calmly and coherently about moral norms and is able to give good reasons for adopting or rejecting such norms. Based on personal reflection, she arrives at conclusions about her own moral code. This person is the 'true individualist', the person who holds true moral autonomy, and, as such, represents the professional ideal (Taylor 1975, p. 10).

As a nurse, one is a member of the society that is nursing. Through a process of education and socialisation, she learns what it is to be a nurse and, like a member of any society, learns and adopts the behaviours, norms, standards and practices of that society, including the moral. These are usually encased in tradition, in authority, and in personal values and beliefs of various nurses with whom she comes in contact. A moral system or perspective can be viewed as a kind of continuum, with ethical egoism at one pole and pure altruism at the other, both representing the extremes of classifications of such systems. A system of ethical egoism holds that self-interest is the sole vital standard of right conduct; it is the good of the moral agent herself, the decision-maker, that is the prime consideration when facing moral issues and dilemmas. In contrast to this ethical egoism is the traditional and customary ethical norm for nursing: the ethic of pure altruism. This holds that the moral ideal for the agent is to 'devote himself to the welfare of others at whatever cost to his own interest' (Taylor 1975, p. 61).

The logic of this is clear when one considers that nursing is essentially a profession founded on the need for care which is based on the value of altruism. It is altruism that allows and even requires that the nurse hold the health and wellbeing of patients in high regard. Because ethical egoism is hardly an appropriate ethical norm for any profession, and pure altruism negates the person who is nurse, it is concluded that both are representative of a customary morality; neither approach considers the consequences to *all* those who are affected by a given ethical decision and great harm can result as a consequence. The moral practice of nursing demands that the nurse adopt a reflective morality in that practice. Through a reflective morality, the nurse can achieve the balance between ethical egoism and pure altruism that is the ethic of practice so essential in professional nursing.

The reflective nurse

Why is critical reflection so important? To paraphrase Stephen Brookfield (1995) in his discussion of critical reflection and teaching, it is important because it helps us take informed actions and develop rationale for practice.

'Critical reflection embeds not only our actions but also our sense of who we are as teachers (nurses) in an examined reality.' (p. 22)

It grounds our most difficult decisions in core beliefs, values, and assumption. Reflective practice is grounded in the idea that we can stand outside ourselves and come to a clearer understanding of what we do and who we are by freeing ourselves of distorted ways of reasoning and acting (p. 214). This becomes the challenge to the reflective nurse: to stand outside herself in a process of discovery in order to come to a clear understanding of what is the essence of nursing, the meaning of her experience, and who is this person who is nurse, as well as to examine critically the theoretical foundations of ethics. This approach represents a new call for the:

'integration of reason and emotion, the personal and the political, the public and the private. In moral theory ... this is part of a general effort to reverse the segregation of intellectual inquiry from personal experience in moral deliberation.' (Lauritzen 1996, p. 6)

He goes on to caution that to offer one's experience as truth is not to claim truth 'with a capital T'. Rather, it is a starting point, not at the end but the beginning of moral deliberation, requiring a critical assessment of experience to uncover meaningful patterns leading to clear and accurate interpretations.

Carper, in her article Fundamental Patterns of Knowing in Nursing (1978), cites personal knowledge and ethics as two of these patterns. These form the crux of reflective practice and are the essential requisites of the reflective nurse. There are two stages or processes of reflective morality, the first consisting of theoretical learning and personal exploration, the second the moral deliberation when confronting a specific moral dilemma or problem requiring judgement and action on the part of the moral agent, the nurse. These two are characterised by the questions of, 'What I ought to *be* and then, 'What I ought to *do*' in order to practice with a reflective morality. There is an ongoing process of reflection on the part of the nurse addressing such questions and issues as: What does it mean to be a nurse? To be moral? What are my values? Why? Are these values conducive to ethical practice? What is the basis for my moral beliefs? What is my experience in the ethical practice of nursing? What are my critical incidents as a nurse? What do these mean? What is the meaning of nursing in my life? What ethical decisions have I made in the past? What does 'patient' mean to me? Who am I in the nurse–patient relationship? What does this relationship mean to me? How do I make ethical decisions? What are my stories? What do I believe about nursing? These concerns and their responses form a kind of autobiography of the reflective nurse leading to that personal knowledge: a formulation of what one ought to be and how one lives the moral life as nurse.

Complementary to such personal knowledge is knowledge of theoretical normative ethics, philosophical inquiry into the nature and bases of morality. One of the chief goals of ethics is to construct rational argument in support of moral judgements, rules or standards. Making moral judgements involves the application of moral norms, either a rule of conduct or a standard of evaluation. Normative ethics asks fairly concrete questions relative to right and wrong actions and establishes a system of moral standards and rules by which to judge an action as right or wrong. Likewise, it provides a set of principles by which alternatives of actions may be analysed and decisions can be made. The reflective nurse has theoretical knowledge of normative ethics; she is able to reflect on ethics principles and concepts incorporating such knowledge into her ethical decision-making process, thereby employing rational delibera- tion in her analysis of ethical issues and moral dilemmas.

The personal and moral sense of nursing are joined together in the nurse–patient relationship (Bishop & Scudder 1990); the person who is nurse and the person who is patient come together as strangers for a specific purpose, in meaningful engagement. It is the nurse who is in the unique position of knowing the person who is patient and, therefore, is able to assist patients in reflecting on the meaning of their life experi- ences. This is a critical aspect of ethical decision-making. The nurse clearly has the responsibility of assisting the patient in this process for, in considering moral problems from only the perspective of ethics theory, the moral agent fails to incorporate the person who is at the centre, the meaning of the experience, the life and living of that person. In dis- cussing one specific instance in which a patient with severe burns was medically treated against his will, Lauritzen (1996) writes that the conventional analysis of such cases, using ethics principles and concepts, is complete.

> 'Such an analysis is inadequate because it fails to do justice to the enormity of the catastrophe that has befallen Dax. It is not – as the conventional analysis would have it – that Dax's quality of life has changed and we must determine who will judge this diminished quality. Rather, the point is that Dax himself has been destroyed.' (p. 11)

It is this that the reflective nurse must grasp and know; this is why nursing ethics is and must be an ethics of practice rather than simply an applied ethic. An apt description of moral reasoning is offered by Jameton (1984):

> 'Reasoning in ethics requires bringing all one's faculties in a balanced way to bear on the sincere concern for human well-being in general and the meaning of human experience. Being reasonable in ethics is more like having integrity than like being smart.' (p. 155)

This captures the essence of reflective morality.

Doing the right thing

'Reflection in and of itself is not enough; it must always be linked to how the world can be changed.' (Brookfield 1995, p. 217)

Nursing is a practice discipline and it is within such practice that moral issues and dilemmas arise, and it is practice that requires resolution. It is through reflection and analysis that the moral practice of nursing is assured and that personal and professional integrity is maintained. Moral reasoning is at the heart of ethical judgement and, to facilitate this process of doing the right thing, a model of ethical decision-making is helpful. It is through such a process that nursing can move from a customary morality to a reflective morality, thus meeting the moral imperative of nursing, excellent practice. Doing the right thing requires knowledge, reflection, analysis, and judgement, the essential elements of this model. Whitbeck (1996), in her discussion of ethics, using design practice in engineering as her analogy, offers valuable insight into reflection and analysis, fully illuminating the complexity of the problem. She writes:

'The question is not simply how I would evaluate proposed courses of action, but how I go about devising such courses of action. It is not enough to be able to evaluate well-defined actions, motives, etc., because actual moral problems are not multiple-choice problems. One must *devise* possible courses of action as well as evaluate them.' (p. 9)

There is rarely one uniquely correct solution or response to moral problems or any predetermined number of correct responses either. However, some responses may be clearly unacceptable and some solutions better than others, and with different kinds of advantages. She maintains that perhaps the misunderstanding and misrepresentation of moral problems is because most ethics and applied ethics have neglected the perspective of the moral agent.

'To frame moral problems primarily from the vantage point of the judge or the moral critic, rather than from that of the person facing the problem, associates ethics with judgement and criticism.' (p. 15)

This does not allow for consideration of multiple constraints and does not incorporate personal reflection or analysis. A model for ethical decision-making, if it is to be transformative of practice, holds such reflection and analysis as an integral component.

A model of ethical decision-making

This model is a reflective model, defining and describing ethical decision-making as three ongoing processes: reflection and analysis; judgement and action; and justification and reflection. It is designed as a process to undertake when confronting a moral problem or dilemma in practice. Personal knowledge and ethics theory are utilised as the basis and this model presupposes the personal reflection on the part of the nurse necessary for reflective morality. The specific steps of this model consist of the following:

(1) Reflection and Analysis
  (a) Name the problem
    - Describe and define the ethical issue, problem, or dilemma. What is the real issue?
  (b) Examine all the dimensions and constraints of the problem
    - Are there rights and duty involved? Whose? Why?
    - What are the relevant ethical principles?
    - What are the legal and professional aspects?
    - What are the personal values, beliefs, experiences of and meaning to the moral agent? to other relevant persons?
  (c) Identify the decision
    - Whose decision is this to make?
    - Is the decision-maker acting alone or with others?
    - Who will be affected by the decision?
  (d) Design the possible solutions: consider the uncertainties
    - What are all the possible choices of action: options?
    - Are any of these clearly unacceptable?
    - What are the possible good consequences of *each* option to *all* those affected?
    - What are the possible harmful consequences of *each* option to *all* those affected?
    - Reflect on the meaning of each option relative to the life of the moral agent.
  (e) Analyse each option
    - For each option: how much and what kind of *good* and of *harm* will result in the lives of all those affected by the decision, as a consequence of choosing this option?
    - Which option leads to the greatest intrinsic good and the least intrinsic harm for the most people, of those affected by the decision?
(2) Judgement and action
  (a) Decide: choose one option.
  (b) Act on that decision.
(3) Justification and reflection
  (a) Evaluate the decision
    - Using ethics theory, justify the decision and action as the morally right thing to do.
    - Using personal reflection, identify that this decision and action was the morally right thing to do.
  (b) Reflection
    - What is the effect of this decision and action on my life? on all those affected? how am I changed?
    - What might I do differently? What next?

- How does this affect my practice?
- How does this experience fit in my life?
- Consider the uncertainties.

Conclusion

In conclusion, a consideration of the implications for transforming nursing practice through reflective morality is indicated. Accepting the premise that nursing is a moral endeavour and that, because of this, excellent practice is the moral imperative of that practice, it is evident that a reflective morality is appropriate. Lauritzen (1996) discusses the idea of 'reflective equilibrium', John Rawls' well-known method of theory testing in ethics which seeks to arrive at a fit among the best competing moral theories. It is suggested that an appeal to experience be incorporated into this 'back-and-forth' process of discussion, analysis and critique, thus using this 'reflective equilibrium' as a process of general moral deliberation (p. 13). Such a process would allow a balance between, and value to, ethics theory and personal knowledge.

Experience is understood as foundational, originating knowledge, not viewed as *truth*, but as *a* truth, *my* truth. This constitutes a beginning of moral deliberation rather than the end point – an 'invitation to discussion', as Lauritzen (1996)) calls it. Such experiences must be drawn together in a meaningful pattern. Further, a reflective morality must take into account and accommodate differences in experience; it must negotiate competing and potentially irreconcilable differences in experiences. This is a challenge.

To utilise experience and meaning as the only path to reflective morality would lead to a kind of moral anarchy, hardly effective for professional practice. Likewise, however, to adopt a rigid adherence to theory and accepted ethics principles would fail to account for the meaning of a moral life, the value of personal experience and knowledge. This too is inappropriate for the moral endeavour that is nursing. It is through reflective equilibrium that practice is transformed; it is this approach that is required if nursing is to move to moral maturity, from a customary to a reflective morality. It is a reflective morality that gives meaning to nursing – to nurses and to those with whom nursing practice is shared, patients. It is this reflective morality that will change the nature of nursing; it is reflective morality that *is* transformational nursing practice.

References

Bandman, E.L. & Bandman, B. (1990) *Nursing Ethics Throughout the Life Span* (2nd edn). Appleton & Lange, Norwalk, CT.

Bishop, A.H. & Scudder, J.R. Jr (1990) *The Practical, Moral, and Personal Sense of Nursing: A Phenomenological Philosophy of Practice.* Suny Press, Albany, NY.

Brookfield, S.D. (1995) *Becoming a Critically Reflective Teacher.* Jossey-Bass Publishers, San Francisco.

Carper, B.A. (1978) Fundamental patterns of knowing in nursing. *Advances in Nursing Science* **1** (1), 3–23.

Engelhardt, H.T. Jr (1986) *The Foundations of Bioethics*. Oxford University Press, New York.

Ferrell, L. (1992) *A dilemma of caring: ethical analysis and justification of the nurse refusing assignment*. Unpublished doctoral dissertation. Adelphi University, Garden City, NY.

Jameton, A.L. (1984) *Nursing Practice – the Ethical Issues*. Prentice-Hall Inc., Englewood Cliffs, NJ.

Lauritzen, P. (1996) Ethics and experience: the case of the curious response. *Hastings Center Report*, **26**(1), 6–15.

Purtilo, R.B. & Cassel, C.K. (1981) *Ethical Dimensions in the Health Professions*. W.B. Saunders Co., Philadelphia.

Taylor, P.W. (1975) *Principles of Ethics: An Introduction*. Wadsworth Publishing Company, Belmont, CA.

Whitbeck, C. (1996) Ethics as design: doing justice to moral problems. *Hastings Center Report*, **26**(3), 9–16.

Yarling, R.R. & McElmurry, B.J. (1986) Rethinking the nurse's role in 'Do not resuscitate' orders: a clinical policy proposal in nursing ethics. In *Ethical issues in nursing* (ed. P.L. Chin). Aspen Systems Corporation, Rockville, MD.

Chapter 4

Nursing as Caring Through the Reflective Lens

Anne Boykin

Introduction

Assumptions underlying the practice of nursing reflect values and beliefs. They direct the perspective of the discipline and therefore significantly influence what is seen and experienced or not seen or experienced. For example, what is seen will be different if the focus for practice is on knowing and nurturing wholeness rather than on particular aspects of the person such as biological or psychological. The views on reflective practice embedded in this chapter emanate from the theoretical framework of *Nursing as Caring: A Model for Transforming Practice* (Boykin & Schoenhofer 1993). The relationship of this nursing practice perspective to reflective practice, and to story as a method for knowing nursing, is described.

Context for reflective practice

Nursing as caring offers a perspective in which both language and intention centre around caring. The fundamental assumptions include:

● to be human is to be caring (Roach 1987)
● personhood is a process of living grounded in caring
● the capacity for personhood can be nurtured through relationships with others
● persons are whole in the moment, growing from moment to moment.

The first assumption is based on Roach's (1987) work which states that all persons are caring by virtue of their humanness. Commitment to this belief fundamentally grounds and establishes the ontological and ethical basis on which nursing as caring is built.

'If the ontological basis for being is that all persons are caring and that by our humanness caring is, then I accept that I am a caring person.' (Boykin & Schoenhofer, 1993, p. 6)

Certain obligations result from this belief, such as a commitment to know self and other as caring. Each person, throughout life, grows in their capacity to express caring. Caring, therefore, is a process and as such as continually unfolding and is lived moment to moment. Our experiences present opportunities to grow in an understanding of what it means to be human and to live caring.

Our way of being in relationship communicates beliefs and values held dear. It is through our relationships that we come to know self and other as caring and to draw forth caring possibilities. The awareness of self as caring persons assists one to recognise that each person lives caring moment-to-moment, in unique ways, and that each encounter is an opportunity to grow in caring. The importance of knowing self as caring cannot be over-emphasised as one can only understand in another what is understood in self. One must have the courage to honestly know self and to discover within self one's own unique expressions of caring. This process requires genuiness and openness. Mayeroff's (1971) views on how one can know caring are helpful in making an abstract construct more concrete. He states that caring is expressed through knowing, patience, alternating rhythms, courage, honesty, trust, humility and hope.

Personhood is the process of living grounded in caring. It is living out who we are. Personhood means living life in congruence with one's beliefs and values. It means being authentic. Personhood is enhanced through participating in nurturing relationships with others. Nursing involves the nurturing of persons living and growing in caring. The nurse enters the world of the nursed with the *intention* of knowing them as caring person and of nurturing them in the process of living caring.

The belief that persons are whole in the moment expresses respect for the *total* person. Relationships are grounded in responding to the wholeness of others. Wholeness is forever present. What this belief acknowledges is that regardless of changes which occur in a person throughout life – such as becoming more educated or more attuned to oneself through life's experiences – each person is as complete as can be at each moment.

'The inherent value that persons reflect and to which they respond is the wholeness of persons.' (Boykin & Schoenhofer, 1991, p. 9)

The call to which nursing is responding is the desire of persons to be recognised, affirmed and supported as caring person. All of these beliefs find their expression in what is called the nursing situation. The nursing situation is understood as 'a shared lived experience in which the caring between nurse and nursed enhances personhood' (or living grounded in caring) (Boykin & Schoenhofer, p. 24). The uniqueness of this perspective lies in the intention of the nurse to nurture the wholeness of persons as they live and grow in caring. As an expression of nursing, caring is the intentional and authentic presence of the nurse with another. The nurse endeavours to come to know the other as caring person and seeks to understand how that person might be supported, sustained, and affirmed (Boykin & Schoenhofer, 1993, p. 25).

Because of the nurse's desire to know the other as caring person, the nurse intentionally enters the world of another and begins to understand calls for nursing. The nurse, through genuine openness and active patience, hears calls for nursing. These calls are for specific forms of caring that acknowledge, affirm and sustain the other as they live caring uniquely. The nurturing response of the nurse to these calls is unique as it reflects the beauty and wholeness of the individual nurse. The way one expresses caring is inherently grounded in who one is and what one knows. The art of nursing is lived in special and individual ways by each nurse and is influenced by the person's experiences, knowledge and patterns of expression.

Living caring is a reciprocal process. It requires the personal investment of both caring persons – the nursed and the nurse who come to know each other as living caring through a mutual unfolding. Trust and courage are needed for such presence to occur. This mutual process is set in motion when the nurse risks entering the other's world and the other invites the nurse into his/her sacred space. They share a coparticipative relationship in which each affirms and describes the caring that is created in the moment.

Reflective practice

To truly nurse, reflective practice is essential. Schön (1983) in his book, *The Reflective Practitioner*, extensively describes reflective practice and includes in this description knowing-in-action, reflecting-in-action and reflection-in-practice.

The first aspect, knowing-in-action, is a tacit dimension. Tacit knowing refers to the fact that we know much more than can be put into words. From the viewpoint of professional practice, there are many times in nursing practice situations where one simply cannot fully describe how or what one knows. This is tacit knowing-in-action. Each nurse depends on this knowing. For example, every competent nurse recognises certain phenomena – such as symptoms of a disease or a knowing of how a patient is experiencing a particular situation – and yet may not be able to give a complete description of these. The nurse may question within, 'What are the familiar aspects of this situation and what is different?' 'What is my framework for being in this situation?'. This knowing-in-action is somewhat spontaneous.

One may also reflect on practice while on is in the midst of it. This process involves both reflection-in-action and reflection-in-practice. Schön suggests these reflections are built on Model II relationships. In contrast to Model I relating, where the professional is viewed as the expert and therefore makes decisions for others, Model II relating recognises the professional as bringing to a situation special knowledges and skills which can be effective in collaborating with others. In this particular relationship, mutuality and importance of others are valued. Schön states that reflection-in-action consists of 'on the spot surfacing, criticizing, restructuring and testing of intuitive understanding of experience phenomena' (Schön, p. 241). It hinges on the element of surprise. Such reflection shapes the moment and has immediate applicability to practice. The process of reflection-in-action is not time limited. It may occur in minutes, days, weeks or even months depending on the situation of practice. When one reflects in practice, the reflections may, in fact, be quite varied. For example, the nurse may reflect on her feelings on a situation, on the way a situation is viewed or on the knowing applied in the situation.

Schön states that:

'just as reflective practice takes the form of a reflective conversation with the situation, so the reflective practitioner's relation with this client takes the form of literally reflective conversation.' (p. 295)

The nurse recognises that her technological expertise has meaning only in the context of the particular situation. The importance of inter-relationship between the nurse and the nursed becomes clear as both offer their understanding, meaning, knowing and planning in the situation. Since meanings of actions embedded in particular situations may vary, the nurse 'recognizes an obligation to make his own understandings accessible to the nursed' (p. 295) leading to continued reflections.

Reflection-in-action calls for intentional and authentic presence through which the wholeness of being is felt. It involves a way of listening and communicating through which one gives of self. This is different from being attentive, for attentiveness is not inclusive of giving of self. As one listens and enters into the dialogue, 'personal reactions are transformed into a sense of a larger reality which trans-cends likes and dislikes' (Richards 1964, p. 107). Consciousness is raised through this experience adding to the moral basis for being in relationship. Presence heightens one's awareness of the moral nature of things.

To be open and present with another one must let go – free oneself from that which burdens us. In a spiritual sense one is emptied in order to be filled with the treasure of the other. Although another's treasure may not necessarily be valued by the receiver, there is, nonetheless, an openness to the gifts of the other; an openness to know and to receive. Presence requires practice and grows through reflection in action.

Each person prepares to enter nursing situations in their own way. For some, meditation may be the way of finding within self quiet solitude. It may be a word or a phrase which has particular meaning to you and allows you to focus. According to Nouwen, it is in stillness we listen. The solitude of these moments fosters compassion and deepens an under-standing of connectedness with other. It prepares us to hear calls for caring and to live our caring expressions.

'If we keep faith with what we truly hear, at our center, in our ear's ear, we may better serve an ideal of quest and compassion.' (Richards, p. 117)

It is within the context of the nursing situation that reflective practice lives. In nursing situations there may be times when a nurse fails to think about the uniqueness of each situation and may therefore fall into a pattern of rigid, non-person focused actions. By contrast, the nurse practicing reflection-in-action gathers every cue, every hunch, every sign, and drawing on a vast knowledge base, reflects on the meaning of these in each particular situation. The nurse uses multiple ways of knowing – personal, empirical, intuitive, spiritual, and ethical – to create the artistry of the moment. Knowing and trusting the different ways of knowing which exist within us illuminates the beauty of practice. The process of reflective practice is central to this artistry. The nurse as artist is influenced by the repertoire of knowledge, experiences, and stories brought to this new and unfamiliar situation. The nurse recognises that each nursing situation is unique – not like any other even though there may be common aspects. Each nursing situation adds to the richness of the next situation.

The nurse and nursed bring to this lived experience the fullness of their being – their wholeness. It is within the nursing situation that the nurse fully engages in the process of coming to know other as caring person. The focus of the nurse is to nurture the wholeness of other as they live and grow in caring. The nurse draws on the multiple ways of knowing in order to create meaning in this particular situation. Through reflection-in-action, the nurse hears calls for nursing and responds with her unique expressions of caring. These nurturing responses support, sustain and affirm the other.

Reflective practice and nursing stories

The knowing of person is accomplished by being open to knowing and participating in personal stories. Stories are an invaluable means by which we come to know the beauty and wholeness of persons (Boykin & Schoenhofer 1991). Sandelowski (1994) describes story as narrative knowing which is essential knowing for health care providers. Reflective practice is integral to this process. Reflections shape the moment and influence the nurturing response of the nurse. This is beautifully illustrated in the following story.

Connections

I was working in a large teaching hospital, the only RN on the night shift for 34 very ill children. With so many tasks to complete in eight hours, I had already begun to organize and set my priorities according to the Kardex orders. As I listened to the change of shift report, I remember getting a strange feeling in the pit of my stomach when the evening nurse reviewed lab results on Tracy P.

Tall. Strawberry-blonde and freckle-faced Tracy was struggling with the everyday problems of adolescence and fighting a losing battle against leukemia. She had been readmitted to our pediatric/adolescent unit numerous times of the past year, and I'd grown quite fond of her. She rarely had visitors and I admired her courage as she faced the usual battery of tests, chemotherapies and transfusions alone. Some of the nurses even expressed resentment toward her mother for the infrequent visits, even though Tracy never complained.

When I made rounds, Tracy was alone. She looked more pale and tired than I'd ever seen her before. As we chatted and I did my usual 'nursing' things with vital signs and IV adjustments, an unexplained feeling told me her mother should be there. I even felt some resentment toward her mother creep in. 'Tracy,' I asked, 'do you mind if I call your mother tonight?' She looked away, but said it would be OK. I probably should have picked up some cues, but I didn't.

I hurried to finish rounds and dialed the phone, half-expecting her mother to make an excuse not to come. 'I really think Tracy needs you tonight,' I said, after a brief introduction. Tracy's mother had been asleep when I called, but said she would come as soon as she could. When she explained that she was a working single parent with two young children, and lived almost two hours away, I felt humbled and almost sorry I had called. But that feeling persisted and I was relieved when she arrived on the unit about 1:30 in the morning.

Tracy was awake when her mother and I went into the room. I wasn't prepared for the interaction between them. I watched Mrs P. stop about three feet from the end of the bed and stand still. Neither of them said much while I was in the room. I left to answer a call bell and returned perhaps 15 minutes later to find the scene virtually unchanged. The distance and silence made me feel uncomfortable. I felt confused and so helpless; it wasn't at all what I expected between a mother and her dying daughter.

'Mrs P,' I asked hesitantly, 'won't you sit on the bed with Tracy and me?' 'I don't think we're allowed', she said. I closed the door and pulled the curtain around the bed as I replied, 'I think it will be all right. Why don't you sit here and I'll sit on Tracy's other side.' I steered her to the edge of the bed where she sat rather stiffly, looking ill-at-ease. I sat on the other side and began stroking Tracy's arm, talking softly to her. Later, as Mrs P. began to relax, I was relieved to see her reach out to tenderly touch Tracy. I left them alone for a while to make rounds again on the other children.

When I returned to her room, Tracy was drifting in and out of sleep and her mother, still sitting on the edge of the bed, was fighting to stay awake. 'Tracy', I called softly, 'is it O.K. if we lie down on the bed with you?' She opened her eyes and nodded. I shifted Tracy's thin body over to make more room for her mother, then lay down beside her on the opposite side of the bed.

Over the next hour or so, the three of us lay together talking quietly. Though she was drifting in and out of a sleep-like state, Tracy roused occasionally to ask a question or comment about something on her mind. At one point, she asked, 'Gayle, why are my feet and legs feeling tingly and falling asleep?' Well, having seen the movie *Coma* just a few nights before, I of course, considered myself an expert on that subject. I smile now as I remember giving her some lengthy explanation regarding oxygen deprivation and carbon dioxide accumulation due to poor circulation. Anyway, she seemed satisfied with my rambling and fell back asleep.

I left them alone for a while to attend to my other mounting responsibilities. The medical intern, having been wakened by another call, inquired about her vital signs. 'I don't know and it's not important right now,' I remember telling him, 'just leave her alone.' I don't know how he knew not to argue, but he did not press the issue and left.

It was close to five in the morning when I returned to the room. Tears came to my eyes as I stood at the foot of the bed and saw Tracy wrapped in her mother's arms, their bodies pressed closely together. Mrs P. lifted her head up from the pillow when I approached the side of the bed to adjust the IV. Tracy felt cool when I touched her arm. I reached for her wrist. There was no pulse and I detected no respirations. My eyes met the gaze of her mother. 'She's gone,' I whispered.

The routine of postmortem care was all too familiar to me – remove IV, identification tags on wrist and toe, body to the morgue within the hour – it all came clearly to mind step by step. Her mother was still looking at me. 'Please don't take her yet,' she pleaded with me, 'please let me stay with her a while longer.' I left the room and closed the door quietly behind me.

It was after 6 o'clock when I slipped back into the room just as the early morning light was coming through the window. 'Mrs P.' I reached out and touched her arm. She raised her tear-streaked face to look at me. 'It's time,' I said and waited. When she was ready, I helped her off the bed and held her in my arms for a few moments. We cried together. 'Thank you, nurse,' she said as she looked into my eyes and pressed my hand between hers. Then she turned and walked away. The tears continued down my cheeks as I followed her to the door and watched her disappear down the hall.

Gayle Maxwell, RN, MSN (Maxwell 1990)

Conclusion

Stories evolve from reflection on practice. Through the methods of reflection and deliberation, stories are restoried for the purpose of reliving. Such examples from nursing practice stimulate us to think about those nursing situations which are an important part of who we are as nurse. They offer us a range of human experiences and invite us to enter them in personal ways. Nursing stories serve as 'an exquisite source for understanding the content of nursing' (Boykin & Schoenhofer, p. 246). They help intuitive thinking grow out of practice and therefore one may be able to make explicit tacit knowing. As nursing practice is articulated, understandings increase and new knowing is generated.

Study of the artistic expressions visible through the medium of story bring to life the meaning of nurse as special artist and nursing as art. It is 'in the realm of the aesthetic, the nurse is free to know and express the beauty of the caring moment … it is this full engagement within the nursing situation that the nurse truly knows caring in nursing' (Boykin & Schoenhofer, 1993, p. 21).

'Nursing is an art; and if it is to be made
   an art,

it requires as exclusive A devotion, as hard
A preparation, as any painter's or sculptor's
Work;
for what is the having to do with dead
canvas or cold marble,
compared with having to do with the living
body – the temple of God's spirit?
It is one of the Fine Arts;
I had almost said,
the finest of the Fine Arts'

Florence Nightingale (Nightingale 1946)

References

Boykin, A. & Schoenhofer, S. (1991) Story as link between nursing practice, ontology, epistemology. *Image*, 23, 245–8.

Boykin, a. & Schoenhofer, S. (1993) *Nursing as Caring: A Model for Transforming Practice*. National League for Nursing, New York.

Maxwell, G. (1990) Connections. *Nightingale Songs*, POB 057563, West Palm Beach, FL.

Mayeroff, M. (1971) *On Caring*. Harper and Row, New York.

Nightingale, F. (1946) *Notes on Nursing*. J.B. Lipincott Co., Philadelphia.

Richards, M.C. (1964) *Centering*. Weleyan University Press, Connecticut.

Roach, S. (1987) *The Human Act of Caring*. Canadian Hospital Association, Ottawa.

Sandelowski, M. (1994) We are the stories we tell. *Journal of Holistic Nursing*, **12**(1), 23–33.

Schön, D. (1983) *The Reflective Practitioner. How Professionals Think in Action*. Basic Books, New York.

Chapter 5
Voice as a Metaphor for Transformation Through Reflection

Christopher Johns and Helen Hardy

Introduction

'Voice' as a metaphor for transformation through reflection is inspired by the work of Belenky *et al.* (1986). Belenky and her colleagues construed the metaphor of voice to characterise the development of women's ways of knowing through a number of levels from silence to constructed knowledge (Fig. 5.1). Each level can be viewed as a realisation of self. The movement to a new level transcends the previous level as a process of transformation or expanding consciousness to become more fulfilled as a person and as a nurse.

- Silence
- Received knowledge: listening to the voice of others
- Subjective knowledge: the inner voice and the quest for self
- Procedural knowledge: the voice of reason
- Separate and connected knowing
- Constructed knowledge: integrating the voices

Fig. 5.1 Women's ways of knowing (Belenky *et al.* 1986).

Through a number of experiences Helen shared within a guided reflection group, we intend to illustrate how she became empowered and transformed to speak with a different voice, and the impact of this development in realising the meaning of caring within everyday practice. The guided reflection group consists of eight practitioners from different practice settings who have contracted to work with myself as supervisor. We meet for 3 hours each week over 30 weeks, interspersed with a number of theory-based workshops. This is accredited as a 60 credit level 3 course within the framework of a BA Healthcare degree and the ENB Higher Award [ENB A29]. The practitioners share their reflected experiences with the supervisor who facilitates learning through experience. Within the text, Helen's words are in a smaller typeface.

Empowerment

Empowerment is the sense of freedom to do something significant in changing one's life. Greene (1988) noted:

> 'To become [different] is not simply to will oneself to change. There is the question of being *able* to accomplish what one chooses to do. It is not only a matter of the capacity to choose; it is a matter of the power to act to attain one's purposes. We shall be concerned with intelligent choosing and, yes, humane choosing, as we shall be with the kinds of conditions necessary for empowering persons to act on what they choose.' (p. 3)

Reflection is used to penetrate the deep embedded conditions of practice that stifle this freedom in Helen's practice. Reflection helps her to understand the meaning of practice necessary for seeing and responding to practice in new ways. Her commitment to practice, already strong, is nurtured and focused as the conditions necessary for empowerment to act on these new understandings. Kieffer (1984) studied the process of empowerment among community leaders in the USA. He noted how this empowerment process involved: 'Reconstructing and re-orientating deeply engrained personal systems of social relations. Moreover they confront these tasks in an environment which historically has enforced their political repression, and which continues its active and implicit attempts at subversion of constructive change.' (p. 27)

Empowerment was the movement from passivity, the perception of self as powerless, often reflected in uncertainty and aggression, towards becoming assertive, able to take confident action considering self's and others' needs. Kieffer's words help Helen to see that empowerment is empowerment against an existing order of things and likely to be resisted by others where their own interests may be compromised. The lived manifestation of empowerment is assertion.

Silence – finding a 'voice'

Silence was an expression of one way of knowing identified within a study of women's ways of knowing by Belenky *et al.* (1986). It is an extremely impoverished way of self-expression. Helen is a staff nurse working on an adolescent orthopaedic ward. Her relationship with doctors was a significant focus for her reflection. She noted:

> Initially, when I reflected on experiences I recall feeling downtrodden by doctors and undervalued by other members of the multidisciplinary team. I identified a need to become assertive. By reflecting on situations that exposed my lack of self confidence, I was able to become more in tune with my feelings.

I gained self-esteem and felt able to voice my opinions. I have been able to develop the skills to effectively communicate with the medical profession and so make desirable practice more of a reality. As an assertive person I feel I am of much greater use to the patients and my colleagues. Conflicting ideas and beliefs are present in health care, and learning to respond effectively in such situations is challenging. Prior to incorporating reflection into my practice I found that the easiest way to deal with conflict was to accommodate another professional's opinions. However, as my self esteem increased, so did my desire to assert my beliefs. I felt I was doing myself no favours by merely agreeing with another professional. I believe that managing conflict effectively stimulates an exchange of ideas which ultimately enhances patient care.

After experiencing a number of situations where doctors ignored what I had to say, my relationship with them became a focus for my reflection. The difficulty I had giving feedback to doctors was complicating my practice. I lacked confidence in entering a discussion with a doctor, yet felt frustrated when he or she did not recognise my experience. Most importantly, I felt that patient care was affected. My integrity was compromised. Yet I also realised, in the interests of my patient, that I needed to work towards developing collaborative relationships with doctors (Keddy *et al.* 1986) rather than marginalising myself as 'stroppy'.

How is it that nurses have been socialised to have no voice in such situations? Do they perceive themselves as subjected to professional dominance by medicine as many authors have suggested (Friedson 1970; Buckenham & McGrath 1983; Hughes 1971; Capra 1982; Brunning & Huffington 1985). Indeed the weight of evidence cannot deny this history. Why have educational processes failed to pay adequate attention to social forces that stifle nurses' voices? Is this a projection of teachers' own lack of voice? A perceived sense of subordination is a major barrier for nurses to realise their desirable beliefs and values as everyday practice (Johns 1994). Helen's experience with Jack illustrates this well.

I suspected Jack had dislocated his hip. As the incident occurred at the weekend I informed the doctor on call. I explained my concerns to him, yet he felt the leg looked in a good position. This doctor did not know Jack at the time and I felt his observation had been insufficient. However, I did not question his judgement or knowledge about the patient. I felt even more frustrated when I subsequently discovered that Jack's hip had indeed dislocated and he would require further surgery to correct this. On reflection, I realised that I did not communicate my observations about Jack's hip in a direct way. I hoped that the doctor would interpret my concern and engage in further discussion about Jack. The doctor failed to pick up my non direct cues and I lacked the confidence to further pursue my concerns. Stein (1978) describes the doctor–nurse game in which the nurse shows initiative and offers significant recommendations, yet appears passive, thus ensuring the doctor's dominance. This is exactly what I had attempted to do in the incident involving Jack. Throughout my professional training I was not encouraged to speak out in the presence of doctors. I was conditioned into a subservient role, powerless to take independent action. I realised that I did not enjoy playing the doctor–nurse game, it was just something I had become accustomed to playing. The game did not enrich my practice. In fact, I saw indirect communication as a barrier.

In contrast, some months later, I confronted a team of doctors about their inappropriate decision to discharge Roxanne. I was concerned that the doctors were being too hasty and explained that Roxanne had only just got her brace [following a spinal fusion] and that she had not slept in it or been seen by either the physiotherapist or occupational therapist. The senior registrar turned to me with an indignant look on his face and asked why it was taking so long to get the patients ready for discharge? On reflection I recognised the open disagreement between myself and the registrar. I had felt embarrassed and saw these feelings as a consequence of not playing the game outlined by Stein. However, I was asserting my voice as I felt it was wrong to let Roxanne think she could go home when her rehabilitation had hardly begun. I realised that although being assertive is an important aspect of giving feedback, the strategy one employs to stimulate discussion is equally important. I wanted to be involved in the decision made about Roxanne's discharge and would have preferred to openly discuss this issue with the doctors. In the past, incidents have occurred when I avoided conflict with a doctor mainly because I saw myself in a no-win situation. With Roxanne's doctors I confronted them in a forthright way. I believe they disapproved of my direct manner and sought to reassert their power by undermining me.

Stein (1978) talked of 'hell to pay' when nurses did not play the game. Chapman (1983) has highlighted how doctors use humiliation techniques to assert the status quo with nurses. Collaboration, whilst an ideal position to work towards, suggests the co-operation of both parties. The assertion of nurses will otherwise lead to 'competitive' modes of managing conflict as the nurse asserts her position against the power interests of the doctor. Johns (1994) states 'despite mutual recognition by both nurses and doctors that the focus of work should be collaborative towards meeting the patient's needs, the reality is that such issues become clouded in professional concerns about power and control'.

By taking the 'moral high ground' of patient interest, based on my unique knowledge about the whole patient, I was able to challenge the power-invested interests of doctors. What I have to learn is not to be intimidated by inappropriate humiliation.

Helen's experiences with doctors reflect her growth from silence to assertiveness. She illustrates reflection as expanding consciousness, moving beyond previous ways of responding to doctors towards new, more desirable and effective relationships. The moral high ground is caring. It cannot be denied, yet it needs to be known.

Received knowledge: listening and speaking with the voice of others

'Women conceive themselves as capable of receiving , even reproducing knowledge from the all knowing external authorities but not capable of creating knowledge of their own.' (Belenky *et al.* 1986)

The practitioner who responds from the position of received voice views the world in a rigid, unimaginative and narrow way. Ways of responding are prescribed rather than interpreted. Intuition is stifled and with it the necessary critical skills to interpret received knowledge creatively and imaginatively within the context of each complex clinical moment. Received knowledge is generally abstract and the philosophy of its construction assumes that such knowledge can explain and predict the world, and as such can be applied within any situation. Such knowledge disassociates theory from practice as two distinct types of knowing. Yet, because it is abstract, it assumes that persons can be reduced to objects to be manipulated. This is the mode of the technician: to follow the rules and to be internally regulated by the rigidity of rules. At this level nurses are not capable of caring.

Subjective knowledge

'The move away from silence and an externally oriented perspective on knowledge and truth eventuates in a new conception of truth as personal, private, and subjectively known or intuited ... what we are calling subjective knowing.' (p. 54)

Belenky *et al.* describes this as the quest for self, for the practitioner to know who she is, the attitudes and beliefs she holds, the concern she feels, the extent to which she knows herself, these are the major points that determine the care she can offer to her patients and families. The focus on self within the context of the clinical or caring moment is the milieu of guided reflection. Reflection honours the self at the centre of caring. It acknowledges who I am as significant and the fears I have as valid. It takes me on a journey that acknowledges my prior experiences as significant. It creates the potential for each moment to be meaningful, and the opportunity to expand my consciousness in caring ways. It takes my fragile commitment and makes it bloom.

Consider Helen's subjective voice:

The type of relationship I form with a patient has always been important to me as I believe that it holds the key to satisfying practice. As a reflective practitioner I have become more interested in the complexities of the nurse–patient relationship and now view my potential to provide care differently. Fundamentally, I now focus on knowing the patient rather than solely concentrating on the issues concerning their hospitalisation. Becoming involved with a patient is often complex, so I used reflection to look more critically at the type of relationship I was forming. I learnt that forming a mutual relationship offered the greatest scope for practice. However, I believe individualised patient-centred care is important and feel this is only available within a holistic framework. To develop a relationship that was holistic required knowing the whole person (Johns 1994). Benner and Wrubel's (1989) work gave me a new insight about my potential to provide care. In practical terms I feel that knowing a person will enable me to effectively help them cope with both health and illness.

Claire

Claire was recovering from a spinal fusion. The incident occurred during a night shift while I was taking my break. Claire was incorrectly moved by an inexperienced agency nurse. Claire subsequently became distressed and was crying in pain. My response to this situation was one of anger. I was upset that the nurse had moved Claire when I had previously explained to her the need for caution during the handling of patients following spinal surgery. I felt responsible as I was Claire's named nurse and knew that she trusted me. I assumed that Claire blamed me for what had happened and tried to reassure her by promising that the nurse would not move her again. In my reflective diary I summed up my anger with the words, 'professional incompetence'.

By reflecting on this experience, I became aware that my angry response was influenced by my protective feelings towards Claire. I blamed myself for her distress. I shared this experience in a group meeting and was challenged by my supervisor who wanted to know if I had actually asked Claire how she felt following the incident. I did not have an answer to his question as I had not encouraged Claire to discuss her feelings. My believe that she thought I had let her down was purely speculative. I struggled to deal with my own feelings of anxiety and cut myself off from Claire's feelings. I have been able to relate much of what Hall (1964) says about 'stewing in one's juices' as being non-productive. Literally this is what I had been doing ever since this situation, feeling angry but unable to deal adequately with the conflict. On reflection, this experience has increased my self awareness that my emotions will profoundly affect my response to a situation. To be effective in a relationship I need to know myself. Only then will I be available for the patient.

Ramos (1992) highlights a nurse's endeavour to imagine a patient's feelings. In such situations Ramos' research showed that a nurse dominated and controlled the relationship. However, Ramos emphasises that this stage could pass and allow a deeper bond to form. In my experience with Claire I felt very much in control of our relationship, which I believe added to my protective feelings towards her. Morse (1991) has characterised the types and analyses the development of relationships. I felt that Claire and I had many of the characteristics that contribute to what Morse would define as a 'mutual connected relationship'. For example, I liked to involve Claire in decisions about her care. However, my professional perspective of Claire was therapeutic. Morse states, 'In the therapeutic nurse–patient relationship, the nurse views the patient first within the patient role and second as a person with a life outside'. I was Claire's nurse and she was my patient, and in this incident I was primarily concerned for her safety. By reflecting on this experience I can see how I also could have addressed Claire's personal needs and not merely tried to reassure her that the agency nurse would not move her again. Following this experience I became more aware of the different aspects that make up a relationship. In addition to knowing myself, I also wanted to know the person behind the patient.

Helen confronts herself with her limited perception of caring. Her concern cannot be doubted but it is misplaced within this limited perception. She begins to articulate a new understanding informed by both her knowing in practice and extant knowledge that informs her and offers a framework for reflection.

Procedural knowledge

'People who experience self as predominantly separate tend to espouse a morality based on impersonal procedures for establishing justice, while people who experience the self as predominantly connected tend to espouse a morality based on care.' (Belenky *et al.* 1986, p. 102)

There are basically two modes of being within procedural knowing: the separate and connected knower. The development of both the separate and connected voice is the explicit focus of reflective practice. Each are important voices, although the connected voice is the crux towards understanding the experience of the other through empathy. Yet it is necessary that the practitioner can draw on and appropriately use theory to inform her practice.

The separate knower becomes adept at criticising the voices of others, what Belenky *et al.* describe as the 'doubting game'. This is an important attribute to use knowledge in a meaningful way, through critique and juxtaposition with personal knowing gained through experience. Such knowledge is then available to be assimilated within personal knowing within the context of the caring moment. The aesthetic response (Carper 1978) – to grasp and interpret the patient's experience, and envisage what might be for the patient – is the essence of empathy. It is only through knowing the patient at this deep level that appropriate caring interventions can be made. This is the caring dance, hopefully a dance that is beautifully choreographed and individually expressed, but also a dance informed with appropriate actions, and techniques informed appropriately by science. It is informed moral caring or praxis. Hence reflection offers a way to synthesise the separate and connected knowers.

Helen continues her story:

This experience took place some months later. Ann had been admitted for an arthrogram of her right hip. Ann was a tom-boy. She hated the pop group Take That, whom the two girls in the bed space either side of her loved, and who were playing their latest video when Ann arrived on the ward. Immediately I sensed that Ann was uncomfortable in her new environment and offered her the opportunity to move into a different bed space. Ann ignored me and her mother said, 'It takes a while for her to settle in'. I was concerned about Ann and decided to pursue forming a relationship. I asked Ann about her hip and knee pain, and how her injury had occurred, but she was still reluctant to talk to me. Her hobbies were football and riding her bicycle. I asked her if her pain restricted her hobbies and she replied 'a bit'. I felt frustrated and wondered what was bothering this young person. I decided that it would be best to give Ann some space, and observed her during the afternoon. When I spoke to her later that evening, she still seemed totally disinterested in me. The following morning when Ann was scheduled to go for her hip arthrogram she became very distressed and abusive. Clearly under that undemonstrative exterior was a frightened young woman I knew nothing about.

I had rarely experienced such a negative response when trying to form a relationship with a patient. My head was buzzing with ideas about gaining her confidence. I wanted to know what she was feeling, and what was bothering her and why she appeared not to like me. When I reflected on this experience I felt very despondent. However, when I discussed this experience with my supervisor I realised that I had been focusing on knowing Ann as a patient rather than as a person. Morse (1991) makes the point about knowing the patient as a person first in a connected relationship. However, I had not shown any particular interest in Ann's hobbies or her life outside of hospital. I did not engage her in any conversation other than that associated with her treatment. I had assumed Ann would want to get to know me; however, she was unwilling to play my game. The more I tried to accommodate her, the more she evaded me. This experience taught me that not all patients welcome a mutual relationship. I was reminded of Hall's observation (1964) that, 'It is impossible to nurse any more of a person than that person allows us to see'. Ann hadn't shown me 'who she was' and I hadn't found out.

Much of the literature about knowing the patient refers to the notion of 'clicking' (Morse 1991; Fosbinder 1994; May 1991). Clicking is defined by Fosbinder (1994) as 'an immediate rapport between patient and nurse'. Morse (1991) suggests that clicking with a patient evokes the development of a deeper relationship. However, there is little literature that discusses the relationship that does not click. From my own experiences these relationships are often much more complex, and require a different approach, one that involves giving the patient space to make contact in their own time rather than imposing myself on them. May (1991) explores neutrality and involvement in nurse–patient relationships. In this study May discusses the benefits of knowing the patient not merely in a clinical sense, but also in a social sense. He suggests that 'reciprocity' is a valuable way to access a person's character. In a number of previous experiences I have found that sharing information about my life outside the hospital has enhanced a relationship. In my experience with Ann it is interesting to speculate how she would have reacted had I shared some information about my social life with her. I feel it would have changed the focus of conversation away from her treatment. I certainly intend to look more closely at different ways of stimulating an interaction with patients who want to reject me.

This experience with Ann taught me that while I still need to focus my mind on knowing the person, I also need to be aware of individual needs: different strategies work for different people. Having this knowledge will enhance my ability to be effective.

Constructed knowing

'Women view all knowledge as contextual, experience themselves as creator of knowledge and value both subjective and objective strategies for knowing.' (Belenky *et al.* 1986).

Constructed knowledge is the successful juxtaposition of all extant sources of knowledge with knowing in practice. Then the person truly speaks with an informed, passionate, subjective voice. It is the voice of wisdom and the voice of the soul. It is a dynamic voice, always expanding in light of new understandings. The final part of Helen's story glimpses her move towards this knowing:

> When I went to admit Angela it struck me that I was clutching her medical notes and nursing documentation. As I sat down next to her, I left these files at the end of her bed and focused my attention on her as a person. The first 15 minutes of our conversation centred on Angela's journey to the hospital and life in her first year at university. Our discussion progressed to the reason for Angela's admission and feelings about her treatment. Finally I turned to the nursing documentation and decided I had obtained more information about Angela then I would have if I had been bound by the constraints of the ward admission tool.
>
> I believe that Angela and I formed a mutual relationship. We clicked and enjoyed sharing information about our life outside the hospital. When I admitted Angela, the ward was not busy and I chose to spend more time with her. Time constraints are often seen as a barrier to effective practice and I appreciate that the demands on staff are usually much greater. However, I believe that spending an extra 10–15 minutes getting to know a person is an effective use of time because understanding them will enhance my ability to provide care.
>
> My philosophy for practice now encompasses that art of knowing the patient as a person first. With this belief firmly fixed in my mind I have decided to utilise the concept of 'knowing the person' within a model of practice. The Burford NDU Model: Caring in Practice, is a reflective and holistic nursing model (Johns 1994) that aims to 'tune' the practitioner into the Unit's philosophy for practice within each clinical moment.

Helen's voice of a constructed knower is imbued with her passion and excitement. The constructed knower lives her praxis, seeking new ways to realise caring horizons. Models of nursing are merely heuristic vehicles on this journey.

In her conclusion, Helen notes:

> Johns (1995) states: 'Reflective practice can be interpreted as being the practitioner's ability to access, make sense of and learn through work experiences to achieve more desirable, effective and satisfying work.' Reflection has enriched my practice and enabled me to develop new skills. It has enabled me to unlock some dilemmas and confront the barriers that impede my practice. This takes an enquiring mind because a practitioner must be ready to challenge their actions and develop new ideas. I no longer feel defeated by the constraints of management and resources, nor do I view myself as a 'mere' staff nurse. I have gained an inner sense of purpose and desire to provide effective care. The no-man's land between reality and desirability have decreased as I continue to face new challenges that arise in my work.

Conclusion

Helen's experiences with the doctors, Claire, Ann and Angela are transformative as she comes to see herself differently through these experiences. Helen highlights an honesty and humility in doing this, illustrating how guided reflection can create a trusting and intimate learning milieu where practitioners can feel safe and loved enough to face who they truly are. As Milton Mayeroff (1971) eloquently says:

> 'Since I do not pretend to be what I am not, I am not humiliated by having others see me truly. The [nurse] who cares is genuinely humble in being ready and willing to learn about the other and her-self, and what caring involves.' (p. 29–31)

The development of her 'voice' marks the passage of transformation. Reflection nurtures the commitment to practice. As Helen noted, 'As my self-esteem increased so did my desire to assert my beliefs'.

It is a positive cycle of expanding consciousness. Reflection has guided Helen to pay attention to the meaning of her practice. In doing so she is challenged to realise her beliefs in everyday practice. This involves confronting contradictions and taking action to resolve these contra-dictions. As she comes to know and realise her beliefs, her commitment is nourished and grows, fuelling the caring endeavour. She becomes increasingly assertive in this knowing. This knowing is an informed knowing, where Helen drew on relevant theory to help her make sense of situations as they arose, and theory that helped her expand her empathic lens to see the patient's situation, yet without prescribing how she should see them. Without doubt knowledge is central to assertion. Within the unique human encounter between Helen and each of her patients, Helen determines the truth of the situation as she perceives it. This truth is not 'outside herself' as something to apply. As Belenky *et al.* have suggested, Helen's perception is based on her empathic knowing of the other. This is the juxtaposition of knowing the other and knowing self fuelled by commitment. It is the synthesis of two simultaneous dialogues – of knowing 'what this experience means to the other' and 'what this experience means to me'.

From a reflective perspective it is important to put Belenky *et al.*'s sense of separate knowing and connected knowing into perspective. Connected knowing is primary and informed by separate knowing. Belenky *et al.* describe the separate knower as a 'doubter', doubting the veracity of what is written for its truth within the particular human encounter. To do less is to diminish the human encounter. The con-nected response is intuitive, a response to the assimilation of multiple forms of knowing in the moment. The intuitive response is reality. It is so complex that it cannot be easily explained. Reflection is a deliberative process of deconstruction in an attempt to understand and learn through the experience with the intent to develop the intuitive response. Such knowing in practice is unique and subjective, mirroring how each clinical nursing situation is always unique and subjective. Constructive knowing is reflexive, continuously expanding though applying and reflection on new situations, a reflection of the practitioner's transfor-mation to realisation of caring in practice.

References

Belenky, M., Clinchy, B., Goldberger, N., & Tarule, J. (1986) *Women's Ways of Knowing*. Basic Books, New York.

Benner, P. & Wrubel, J. (1989) *The Primacy of Caring: Stress and Coping in Health and Illness*. Addison-Wesley, Menlo Park.

Brunning, H. & Huffington, C. (1985) Altered images. *Nursing Times*, **81**(31), 24–7.

Buckenham, J. & McGrath, G. (1983) *The Social Reality of Nursing*. Adis, Sydney.

Carper, B. (1978) Fundamental patterns of knowing in nursing. *Advances in Nursing Science*, **1**(1), 13–23.

Capra, F. (1982) *The Turning Point, Society and the Rising Culture*. Fontana, London.

Chapman, G.E. (1983) Ritual and rational action. *Journal of Advanced Nursing*, 8, 13–20.

Fosbinder, D. (1994) Patient perceptions of nursing care: an emerging theory of interpersonal competence. *Journal of Advanced Nursing*, 20, 1085–93.

Friedson, E. (1970) *Professional Dominance*. Aldine Atherton, Chicago.

Greene, M. (1988) *The Dialectic of Freedom*. Teachers College Press, Columbia University, New York.

Hall, L.E. (1964) Nursing–what is it? *The Canadian Nurse*, **60**(2), 150–54.

Hughes, E.C. (1971) *The Sociological Eye: Selected Papers*. Aldine Atherton, Chicago.

Johns, C. (1994) Constructing the BNDU Model. In *The Burford NDU Model, Caring in Practice* (ed. C. Johns), pp. 20–58. Blackwell Science, Oxford.

Johns, C. (1995) The value of reflective practice for nursing. *Journal of Clinical Nursing*, 4, 23–30.

Keddy, B. *et al.* (1986) The doctor–nurse relationship: an historical perspective. *Journal of Advanced Nursing*, 11, 745–53.

Keiffer, C.H. (1984) Citizen empowerment: a developmental perspective. *Prevention in Human Services*, **84**(3), 9–36.

May, C. (1991) Affective neutrality and involvement in nurse–patient relationships: perceptions of appropriate behaviour among nurses in acute medical and surgical wards. *Journal of Advanced Nursing*, 26, 552–8.

Mayeroff, M. (1971) *On Caring*. Harper Perennial, New York.

Morse, J. (1991) Negotiating commitment and involvement in the nurse–patient relationship. *Journal of Advanced Nursing*, 16, 455–68.

Ramos, M.C. (1992) The nurse–patient relationship: themes and variations. *Journal of Advanced Nursing*, 17, 496–506.

Stein, L. (1978) The doctor–nurse game. In *Readings in the Sociology of Nursing* (eds R. Dingwall & J. McIntosh), pp. 108–17. Churchill Livingstone, Edinburgh.

Chapter 6

Unfolding the Conditions where the Transformative Potential of Guided Reflection (Clinical Supervision) might Flourish or Flounder

Christopher Johns and Brendan McCormack

Introduction

We assume that guided reflection has the potential for transforming nurses and nursing towards realising desirable work in their everyday practice. Yet:

'the word potential rises like a spectre, because like other recent developments in nursing it promises much. Without doubt, the realisation of this promise is dependent on creating the conditions under which it can flourish.' (Johns 1995, p. 29)

In this chapter, we intend to take the lid off guided reflection to gain an understanding of the conditions where it might flourish or why it might flounder.

Context

Our understandings originate from a collaborative study that commenced in 1989 within a community hospital (Johns 1997). The unit practised primary nursing and I wanted to work with primary and associate nurses in ways that could fulfil my self-perceived clinical leadership role of enabling and supporting the staff to succeed in their roles and to construct collegial relationships between myself and staff that were considered necessary to support primary nursing (Manthey 1980). My solution was to establish guided reflection. Hence I became manager, supervisor and researcher. In the autumn of 1991 I contracted guided reflection with six others. Five were managers of clinical practice. Brendan was a clinical lecturer in nursing. This role was established in an attempt to create clinical leadership-educational roles which drew their influence from engaging in clinical work, with a formalised right to influence the clinical environment and make managerial decisions within the service unit.

In establishing these relationships, the deal was that they simultaneously entered into similar relationships with practitioners within their sphere of practice. Hence I supervised their supervision. Brendan also worked within a community hospital with 30 in-patients and 8 day-patients. There was an espoused philosophy based on humanistic beliefs about nursing, but in reality little opportunity was made available for the patients to exercise freedom of choice, take risks, express opinions, make decisions, and be listened to. In other words, everyday practice presented as a contradiction with the espoused beliefs.

By reflection we mean:

'a window for practitioners to look inside and know who they are as they strive towards understanding and realising the meaning of desirable work in their everyday practices. The practitioner must expose, confront and understand the contradictions within their practice between what is practised and what is desirable. It is the conflict of contradiction and the commitment to achieve desirable work that enables the practitioner to become empowered to take action to appropriately resolve these contradictions.' (Johns 1996)

From the outset, it was never assumed that reflection needed to be guided. My subsequent work with practitioners has convinced me that this is probably essential. Besides the technical difficulty of knowing how to reflect and learn through reflection, reflection needs to be guided because practitioners require guidance to see beyond themselves – to see how their own self-distortions and limited horizons, and those forces embedded within practice, have limited their ability to know and achieve desirable work. Practitioners also require high challenge to confront contradiction and high support to nurture and sustain the commitment, courage and effort to resolve contradiction, and transform self as necessary to realise desirable work as everyday practice. The space and time for guidance coincide with the recent interest in clinical supervision. This is a term defined within the Vision for the Future paper (NHSME 1993) as:

'a term used to describe a formal process of professional support and learning which enables individual practitioners to develop knowl-edge and competence, assume responsibility for their own practice and enhance consumer protection and safety of care in complex situations. It is central to the process of learning and to the expansion of the scope of practice and should be seen as a means of encouraging self-assessment and analytical and reflective skills.' (p. 3)

Implementing clinical supervision is one of 12 targets set out in the Vision for the Future document, that NHS Trusts are expected to comply with. The definition of clinical supervision intends various outcomes in which exist an inherent tension between the enabling/supportive function and the quality assurance function. Clearly, what the practi-tioner discloses within guided reflection can be responded to from either or both of these perspectives depending on their own agenda.

This reflection on the transformative potential of guided reflection (or clinical supervision) is structured around the template of 'being available'. It was evident from an analysis of practitioners' shared experience that the practitioner being available to work with the patient and family was the key therapeutic factor for the practitioner to achieve desirable work.

Being available has a number of dimensions that influence the extent to which the practitioner is available in practice. It was evident from an analysis of the dynamics of guiding reflection that the dimensions of 'being available' were equally applicable for understanding the therapeutic relationship between the supervisor and practitioner. Figure 6.1 sets out this parallel pattern. The central role of the supervisor is to work with the practitioner towards achieving their best interests. The parallel pattern of 'working with' is significant on two levels of congruence; firstly that developmental processes need to be compatible with intended outcomes, and secondly the research methods needed to understand these processes need to be congruent with developmental processes.

In unfolding the significance of this template we draw extensively on dialogue taken from Brendan's guided reflection sessions with practitioners. This dialogue is also used to illustrate the reflexive and temporal process and outcomes of guided reflection.

Being available to work with the practitioner towards achieving desirable practice

This requires an understanding of what desirable practice is. We assume that guided reflection requires two people who share a similar vision of clinical practice and supervision. Incompatibility will lead to different agendas and mutual frustration. Reflection-on-experience provides the supervisor with a rich feedback of practitioner performance and effectiveness, although this information depends on the extent of the practitioner's disclosure. If the supervisor intends, or the practitioner believes, that the primary function of supervision is to judge their performance, then they may be reluctant and resistant to disclose experience.

An emphasis on the monitoring performance role smacks of new methods of surveillance, a word ominously close in meaning to the traditional meaning of 'supervision', to produce a docile and competent workforce (Foucault 1979) – indeed the hallmark of bureaucratic systems. If this is so, then what at once promised transformation becomes a powerful vehicle for conformity and control. We believe that within a transformative milieu, practitioners are helped to monitor themselves as part of a process of developing responsibility. By definition, an effective practitioner knows, monitors and ensures their own effectiveness. Indeed the definition of supervision within the Vision for the Future document emphasises this possibility:

Clinical context		Guided reflection context
Concern		Positive regard • Practitioner commitment
Knowing the person		Knowing the practitioner • Creating a climate for disclosure of experiences • Knowing their practice
Responding with appropriate ethical, informed and skilled interventions	Being available to work with the client/practitioner Shared vision	Responding with an appropriate helping style • Balance of challenge and support • Framing perspectives
Knowing and managing self within a relationship		Knowing and managing self within a relationship • Controlling the agenda • Managing own concerns
Creating and sustaining an environment where being available is possible		Creating and sustaining an environment where being available is possible • Practicalities of ensuring frequent continuity supervision • Conducive environment

Fig. 6.1 The parallel pattern of therapeutic work within clinical practice and within guided reflection based on the core concept of 'being available' (Johns 1997).

'It [clinical supervision] is central to the process of learning and to the expansion of the scope of practice and *should be seen as a means of encouraging self-assessment* and analytical and reflective skills.' (p. 3)

So which way does it go? Can there be a balanced view? This can be visualised through mapping a grid based on the twin axes of intent and emphasis and the knowledge-constitutive interests identified by Habermas (1971) (Fig. 6.2).

The axes of intent and emphasis are finely balanced. The supervisor's emphasis is either towards producing the outcome or on the learning

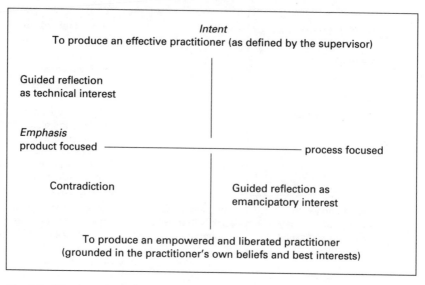

Fig. 6.2 The intent-emphasis axes of guided reflection (Johns 1997).

process. All supervisors I worked with espoused the intent of an empowered and liberated practitioner, although their emphasis in practice was often misplaced. Without doubt supervisors set the pace and tone of the relationship – as might be expected as both parties were coming from hierarchical perspectives. To equalise power takes an active 'letting go' and construction of a new type of relationship. The fact that this was espoused did not mean it existed. In general, the research indicated that the closer line-managers were to practice the more outcome oriented they were as supervisors. Yet it was also evident that a focus on 'outcome' was counter-productive as an effective learning milieu because the practitioner sensed the pressure to perform and change and resisted. The risk is that such relationships lead to a downward spiralling cycle of increased challenge and increased resistance. Being process-oriented always had to be worked towards, as will be apparent within Brendan's reflection.

Brendan's reflection

Practitioners in the clinical area did not always recognise the need for development or the need for improvements in the organisation and delivery of care. Work was merely 'busywork' (Jarvis 1992) centred within a business like routine, with the possibilities that lay within the task itself not being recognised because of the demand for task completion. Whilst I raised people's consciousness of these practice issues, there was little understanding of how changes could be made. The 'swampy lowlands of practice' (Schön 1991) were too swampy and the task ahead insurmountable. On 16 December 1991, I commenced a supervision relationship with Laura, a primary nurse in the unit whom I identified as someone with potential to change and initiate change in others. Indeed she had expressed anger, frustration and exasperation with others' practice but felt powerless to make changes.

Consider this extract from Laura's dairy shared with me in our first supervision session, dated 16 December 1991:

'I find this emphasis on getting through the work so stressful. It affects the way I work with patients. I feel so unhappy at having to leave patients when I have not completed my work with them. There is too much emphasis on morning care in this unit, as most staff work between 9 and 12. This situation is made worse by other staff not carrying out care I have planned. I went away for a weekend and came back to find that one of my patients had developed a pressure sore, and a dressing that I had prescribed 'daily' had not been done at all during my time off. I was so angry and upset, but what could I do? I talked with the person concerned [when I had calmed down] and re-explained the reason for the care plan, but nothing changed. The person seemed to take my feedback all right, but later I heard from somebody else that she was upset about it and was 'bitching' about me to one of the auxiliary nurses.'

For Laura, being available for supervision was yet another factor in juggling time that was not within her control. The emphasis was on completing the tasks within the given time and any new demand on her time, for example giving psychological support and information to relatives were seen as distractions and barriers to effectively achieving her work schedule. Being available, then, was not just about making time for supervision, but instead supervision work needed to parallel changes to the nature of practice itself. That is, making time for supervision needed to fit in initially with a 'task' approach to practice. To suggest that supervision was of more importance would have resulted in even further frustration, as it would have become another new demand on time that prevented effective practice rather than facilitating growth.

To this end, supervision sessions only took place during lunch breaks. Initially Laura could cope with this, as it meant she could create a rigid system of control over the planning of lunch breaks because she 'had to' go to supervision. Often she would miss lunch breaks because of work pressures and this system guaranteed a break every two weeks. While Laura viewed supervision as 'time out', it soon became a 'task' in itself. The challenge for me was to convince Laura that I did understand the practice culture. For Laura, the demonstration of this understanding entailed me operating in a hierarchical mode where I 'told' people what was acceptable and reprimanded those who did not conform – a situation I found intolerable. For a long time, I had to carefully balance collusion with a hierarchy with the facilitation of professional growth.

The current literature suggests that practitioners should choose their supervisor and the type of supervision they require (UKCC 1996). While practitioners who are self aware of their development needs in order to develop therapeutic competence may recognise the need for such supervision, for many this is not the case. Either they do not recognise their own need for such development or they do not know of someone who they feel can meet their needs. In Laura's case, she did not choose her supervisor and indeed, at this particular time, it would have been unrealistic to have expected this. The challenge for me, as the clinical leader with a desire to change practice, was to introduce the concept of reflective practice as a medium for exposition of the values that existed among practitioners and the development of a shared vision. In many respects Laura was used as a 'guinea pig' for this work. Further, the exposition of one practitioner to change without the culture of the organisation changing, places the individual practitioner in an even further challenging situation.

Positive regard

Laura knew that practice had limited therapeutic value due to cultural, attitudinal and organisational factors, and she desperately wanted to change it. Indeed her favourite coping phrase in supervision was 'things will be different when you have made the changes that are needed around here'. This desperate need for change is a reflection of her commitment towards her practice. Being available for supervision requires a commitment to it from both supervisor and practitioner. Practitioners must *want* supervision. It was striking how practitioners' commitment towards supervision was a reflection of commitment towards clinical practice. Just as the practitioner needs to feel positive towards the patient and family, so the supervisor needs to feel positive towards the practitioner. In other words, the practitioner needs to matter to the supervisor. It is the essence of caring, because caring sets up possibilities. The nature of individual reflection is intimate. It is the space where the practitioner discloses self through shared experience, where the practitioner can be known.

Brendan deliberately chose Laura as his first practitioner to supervise because of her positive regard towards her work and her potential to act as a role model to other nurses. Having positive regard for another raises issues about the importance of contracting for supervision. The contract is not just about the setting of ground rules and the explication of possibilities; it is also a time when the supervisor and practitioner articulate their practice beliefs and attitudes and make them available for the other to decide if this person is somebody they can work with. Like any other relationship, choosing one's partner needs to be deliberate and honest.

Knowing the practitioner and their practice

In clinical practice, to use Lydia Hall's (1964) words, 'We can only nurse what the patient allows us to see'; so in supervision we can only guide experience as much as the practitioner allows us to see their experience. The practitioner is known through the experiences they share. Hence the factors that influence disclosure become very significant learning dynamics.

Perhaps the most significant of these dynamics is the practitioner's sense of concern for their practice, given that people will only pay attention to things that matter to them. If someone does not care much for their practice, reflection on experience may well be a chore. In a world where satisfaction is often making it through to the end of the day with minimal hassle, being expected to reflect on and share experience may be galling. Dewey (1936) and Fay (1987) note that a sense of willingness and commitment are pre-requisite to reflection. Therefore, the supervisor may need to spark a dormant sense of commitment in many practitioners who may be burnt-out through working in uncaring environments. It is likely that the types of experience to which practitioners pay attention are those invested with anxiety because they have crashed through sub-consciousness. Hence they are situations of vulnerability.

Brendan knew Laura's practice well. In my role, while I acknowledged the existence of negative beliefs and attitudes, and their effect on patient care, I also recognised the difficulties in changing such attitudes. The realities of equality of need and individuality often posed insurmountable ethical challenges for the practising nurses. Subsequently, nurses found themselves colluding with an institutional environment that tightly scheduled each day's activities within a series of explicit but unwritten rules. The more the supervisor is intimate with the practitioner's practice, the easier it becomes to relate to this practice . On the other hand it becomes less likely the practitioner can escape any intent of surveillance.

Some supervisors were concerned with their self-perception of their clinical credibility. In general it seemed the more removed the supervisor perceived self from practice, for example the district nurse managers, then the more they felt uncomfortable with their supervision ability. This was highlighted with a need to have answers to problems, to be able to 'fix-it' for practitioners, that reflected a socialised position of authority. The other side of this understanding was how the same supervisors felt that practitioners were stressed enough without adding to it through high challenge. These positions reflected a paternalistic attitude that was the antithesis of growth of practitioners into responsibility roles.

Responding with an appropriate helping style

The helping style was reflected within a model of structured reflection (Johns 1995), constructed through reflective cues to enable the practitioner to challenge self and tune into cognitive, affective and temporal processes of learning. Balancing challenge and support in supervision was seen as an essential element of the success of the supervision relationship. The significance of challenge is acknowledged by Blocher (1983), who has set the climate for supervision:

'The supervisor who communicates warmth, respect and genuineness, and positive regard will create a relationship in which the supervisee feels accepted rather than threatened and can be open rather than defensive. In this environment the supervisee can 'hear' straightforward feedback and challenge to risk and grow; the supervisor's main task can then be to monitor the balance of challenge and support in the learning environment.' (Borders & Leddick 1987, p. 47)

This balance of challenge and support unfolded in practice as a delicate affair – excess challenge and we enter a hostile world of threat that prompts defensive flight and fight responses; excess support and we enter a comfortable world. Neither are environments for learning, and yet each world was easy for practitioners and supervisors to slip into. Supervisors who perceived themselves as clinical leaders had strong values about clinical practice. As such, they were always at risk of using high challenge to assert these values in their anxiety to transform practice. Practitioners could only move or be transformed at their own speed. Where practitioners could not move fast enough, this often led to mutual frustration, the perception of threat and a paradoxical breakdown in the learning milieu as supervisors responded with even greater challenge and practitioners recoiled from being hurtled into brick walls of unrealistic expectation. On the other hand, other supervisors felt uncomfortable with challenge because of its connotation with conflict – in a world where people were motivated to avoid conflict. Consider these dynamics within Brendan's dialogue with Laura.

Brendan's reflection

Supervision session 3, 23 January 1992

> **BMc:** How has it been since last session?
> **Laura:** The relationship between me and George that I discussed in the last session has improved although I still do his dressings in the mornings. Anyway I don't want to talk about that today. I've been really annoyed with you all week.
> **BMc:** Why, what did I do?
> **Laura:** You challenged me about May going home because she was still confused. I couldn't believe you did that to me. I felt personally 'got at' by you because you made it look like I didn't know what I was doing. As if I was making a wrong decision. I knew I was taking a risk but I also knew it was the right thing to do.
> **BMc:** Why did you take this challenge personally?
> **Laura:** I had calculated the risk and from my accountability perspective, it was O.K. On the one hand you challenge me to take risks, but on the other hand when I had done so, you were telling me not to!
> **BMc:** Why do you get so annoyed with me for challenging you? Professional challenge should be O.K.
> **Laura:** I knew the patient better than you, and what she was capable of.
> **BMc:** Why take the challenge personally instead of professionally?
> **Laura:** You undermined my knowledge of this patient.
> **BMc:** But Laura, in a different setting a medical consultant would ask such challenging questions of you, and that would be accepted without question.

Why then should a challenge from me, a nurse and colleague, be any different in principle?
Laura: You have more knowledge than me about such situations and you can 'use' that.

Although I made myself available for Laura both in and out of supervision, for her the challenges that she faced were too painful to contemplate. For the majority of supervisees, balancing conformity to the dominant organisational culture with a personal desire for changes created internal conflict. While the supportive component of supervision enables practitioners to develop strategies for dealing with this conflict and the securing of practice changes, for most supervisees the stress caused by 'being seen as different' remains a dominant conflict. Therefore, even the simplest of challenges resulted in a sense of threat and caused her to retreat to old norms. My clinical role legitimised my challenge but often led to such conflicts because of my drive towards accountability for safe and creative practice. While Laura had a similar ambition, the size of the challenge that she alone had come to recognise was too great to contemplate. Therefore, ironically, being clinically credible was not an advantage in this situation as it exposed realities that Laura had little control over. Indeed, in some respects, such credibility was a disadvantage as my position in the organisation meant that I could transcend some of the problems. Being seen to do this further exacerbated the level of frustration experienced by Laura and excused change of action – the 'it's all right for him scenario'.

Because I was focused on achieving an outcome from his work, i.e. changed practice, at times during supervision I used excessive challenge. Through my own supervision with Chris, I grew to recognise that I was using these nurses as agents to bring about change that I desperately wanted. A parallel pattern existed between the realities of practice and the realities of supervision. In practice, the nurses' concern with the organisation interfered with their ability to see the patients' concerns. While in supervision, my concerns about practice interfered with the way I saw the practitioners' concerns and led to my influencing their agenda. Carl Rogers' (1983) notion of authenticity became a significant influence through surfacing my concerns, frustrations and desires at appropriate opportunities. This resulted in me being seen more as a human being with feelings rather than a 'robot with an agenda'. While the role of the supervisor is to support another's reflection, supervisors are human too, and by being authentic I was able to demonstrate my concerns about the feelings of others. This shift in emphasis to the *process* rather than the *product* of supervision paralleled the way practice changes occurred, with the expression of emotion being seen as an important part of showing concern about others.

Framing perspectives

It was evident how the supervisor used a range of framing perspectives to focus and guide reflection on significant aspects of learning. Making these visible offers a checklist to maximise the transformative potential of guided reflection (Fig. 6.3). These perspectives have been evident within Brendan's dialogue with Laura.

- *Framing the development of effectiveness*
  Recognising reflexive learning in adequate ways. This is achieved by practitioners looking back and seeing how they have become changed people in the context of their shared experiences. Templates such as 'being available' help to structure this understanding of learning.
- *Philosophical framing*
  Confronting and clarifying the beliefs/values that constitute desirable practice.
- *Role framing*
  Clarifying role boundaries/relationships/legitimate authority and power within practice.
- *Theoretical framing*
  Assimilating theory and research findings with personal knowing.
- *Parallel pattern framing*
  Acknowledging and exploiting the parallel nature of supervision and clinical practice, for example through role modelling, responding to the practitioner as a person, using catharsis, confrontation, and other intervention skills.
- *Problem framing*
  Posing, clarifying and resolving problems framed within experience.
- *Reality perspective framing*
  Acknowledging the real world and that practising in new ways is not necessarily easy – while helping the practitioner to become knowledgeable and empowered to take necessary action.
- *Temporal framing*
  Recognising that reflection is not an isolated event but connected through experiences over time and anticipating future experiences.

Fig. 6.3 Framing perspectives (Johns 1997).

In the following dialogue with Mary, Brendan pays particular attention to perspective and temporal framing.

Brendan's reflection

Supervision session 18, October 1993 (one year after commencing supervision)

> **Mary:** I want to talk about Susan [her patient]. In the last supervision session, you gave me an exercise to compare the autonomy model with how I practise. I have tried to apply this to my relationship with Susan but somehow it seems different – my relationship with Susan is different and is sometimes inconsistent. I feel I am becoming protective and possessive of Susan. I refused help from Jane [a colleague] this morning because of this.
> **BMc:** Why did you refuse?
> **Mary:** I know how Susan likes to be cared for and her likes and dislikes. I am unsure how other people would view the relationship I have with Susan in relation to autonomy and choice.

Brendan helped Mary explore how she worked with Susan within the autonomy model and her difficulties in getting her colleagues to respond in similar ways. This exposed a culture of conflict avoidance with a consequence of unresolved conflict and poor communication. Supervision gave the practitioner permission to accept her practice shortcomings and the conflicts that existed between her espoused beliefs and her practice reality. There are times when people cannot cope with their own feelings without some assistance. Often Mary would be tearful during supervision as a means of emotional release from the internal conflicts she experienced. Such spilling over of emotion demonstrated Mary's inability to contain her emotions about her practice. Supervision helped Mary to see that feeling like this was not 'abnormal', but indeed the opposite was the case. By having these feelings Mary was demonstrating the essence of a caring relationship, i.e. expressing concern for another. The supervision process channelled these feelings towards humanistic action, thus empowering Mary to attain the confidence to, not just to gain freedom to, change organisational values. By being directed towards appropriate theoretical approaches, Mary learned to articulate her practice values confidently with others.

Knowing and managing own concerns

In Brendan's dialogue with Mary, she chose to talk about Susan. How Brendan picks up cues is inevitably a reflection of points that strike him as significant, and gives him some control of the agenda. Controlling the agenda is a reflection of power interests. We assume that the practitioner needs to dictate the content of supervision, or in other words, to share what she feels appropriate to disclose. Where the supervisor feels the practitioner is avoiding discussing certain aspects of role, this can be noted without challenging the focus for control. It was evident how supervisors who know the practitioner's practice were more likely to feed this knowledge into the supervision session. Again drawing on Hall (1964), just as the practitioner needs to know self and manage self's concerns in order to be available for therapeutic work, so does the supervisor. As Brendan has illustrated, the supervisor may see the practitioner through a haze of their own concerns that blurs the therapeutic potential.

Creating and sustaining an environment where being available is possible

All the foregoing issues contribute to a climate where the supervisor can be available to work with practitioners. Other issues we have not addressed in this chapter concern the practicalities of ensuring adequate continuity of sessions within a conducive environment. Yet can conclusions be drawn about who the supervisor should be? Without doubt supervisors need certain skills. Brendan has illustrated these well through his dialogue. Indeed within the theory of parallel pattern, these skills are those of the effective practitioner. Perhaps most significantly, supervisors need to be perceived as caring.

One influencing factor is how the practitioner might perceive where the supervisor is coming from, in contrast to where the practitioner might want to get to. Where practitioners have been silenced and oppressed – as indeed many nurses socialised within hierarchical-bureaucratic modes of organisation and medical hegemony feel (Roberts 1983) – the idea of being supervised by their manager may be treated with some caution, particularly if they have no choice in this. Yet there are real advantages to being supervised by the line manager (Fig. 6.4) – that may be lost within an emotional rejection of this idea – to the extent of asking, 'Will supervision be less meaningful if not from managers?' In contrast, a number of potential disadvantages in being supervised by line managers were also apparent (Fig. 6.4). Line managers as supervisors could not easily be two separate people. It is interesting to speculate whether people will change their management style to match the supervision style, or whether people will supervise to fit their existing management style. Two ends of a spectrum but which way is it likely to go? Our evidence suggests the latter despite espoused intent to the contrary.

Advantages of manager-supervisor	Disadvantages of manger-supervisor
• Understands the practitioner's practice • Can tackle situations together • Work towards a 'new type' of relationship based on openness and authenticity • Spill-over of supervision work into everyday practice • Mutual growth and empowerment • Work together to realise a shared vision of practice • Opportunity to acknowledge and value practitioners	• Need to 'fix-it' syndrome • Paternalistic – takes action on behalf of the practitioner • Supervises as manages – reinforcing dependency and hierarchy • Conflict over what is best – threat to hierarchical control • Manipulates agenda to suit own needs • Supervision seen as moulding an ideal practitioner or being remedial • Takes on board practitioner's distress • ('Maternal role for hurt child') – cannot detach self from situation • Lack of vision to see other ways of doing things (tainted with the same brush as the practitioner) • Practitioner may avoid sharing certain types of experiences, especially if grounded in inter-personal conflict with the manager-supervisor

Fig. 6.4 The relative potential advantages and disadvantages of line-management supervision.

Brendan's reflection

By April 1993 all team leaders/primary nurses had commenced individual supervision. The hospital manager and I had also commenced peer supervision with each other (McCormack & Hopkins 1995). Although individual attitudes to practice had begun to change, the overall culture of practice had not changed because of the team's inability to share their beliefs and values and challenge each other's practice. Even when challenge did occur, this was often handled in a confrontational way, as this example from Mary's reflective diary illustrates.

'Several days ago, two colleagues related incidents to me which they wanted to raise with another colleague but felt they couldn't. Both had felt upset, angry, hopeless, and a coward because they felt unable to confront the person in question. Both had spent time at home brooding about things. I listened to them, and said that I felt they should be able to talk to the appropriate person. They both felt 'no', they couldn't do this; they were frightened of being shot down, being made to look small. I explained that we are trying to move away from a culture of 'bitching' to one where challenge was accepted in practice.

On reflecting upon this, I realised that rather than forming therapeutic teams, we have harmonious teams (Johns 1993), where we try and cover up the cracks. There will be conflict in a therapeutic team, but this is accepted as part of the process of learning to engage in purposeful and supportive relationships. Now we are aiming to be more therapeutic and collegial, I don't want this any more. I feel I've been evading this issue for long enough. I feel quite strongly about it and everything I am preaching is a sham if we don't address this! Yet I too sometimes go home feeling 'the pits' – low, hopeless, and unable to change. If I feel this bad at being unable to question, how much worse do the primary and associates feel?'

Mary's words represented the growing recognition for all of us to meet as a reflective group, in order to share challenges, issues and developments, with the agenda to transform our ways of relating to each other to what Argyris and Schön describe as model 2 behaviour (1989) ; with its emphasis on open communication networks, where ideas are shared and practice is constructively challenged; where focused development leads to the emancipation of individuals through an increased internal commitment; where there is an emotional self-awareness among team members with freedom to express feelings and an overall interdependence among team members.

Despite the intention to move to model 2 ways of relating with each other, it was not until three years later that members of the group could begin to identify that this was actually realised in practice. The time span reflects the latency of this change process, highlighting how embodied ways of relating are not easy to change. In the group supervision session in April 1996, I prompted the following reflections by Lisa and Cathy.

Lisa: I am now able to recognise and acknowledge my own skills that I have. I feel confident and comfortable with these and am aware of the areas where development is needed. I feel more like a team leader because I have come through a process. I feel more able to recognise others' points on the same journey and that can vary. I can recognise who was significant in helping me and can recognise that in times of difficulty during that development I wasn't abandoned or ignored. I can feel the warmth of the other person, see their anxiety, and can balance this against my own expectations of them in the short term, to enable growth to occur. In recognising how far you can take them, it is important not to lose sight of the beginning of that journey and their starting point.

Cathy [primary nurse]: I can identify with others' feelings and in doing this, I can challenge them when I see them practising in a way that goes against our agreed philosophy. I have a sense of commitment to the journey that is being created and because of this experience a sense of belonging. It's O.K. now to make mistakes, to laugh, and not be serious, to enjoy myself at work and to cry if I need to. I feel an inner strength that guides my action. When Dr Jones came to the unit last week I felt he was avoiding me. I felt this may have been because of a problem with a fax. I decided to approach him and asked him if he was avoiding me? He said he wasn't, but then asked me if he had got me into trouble because of the mistake with the fax. I then knew that his non-approach was related to his feelings of embarrassment. My confidence to approach the doctor in this way demonstrates the growth that has taken place within me. The honesty that has existed in supervision has been transferred into practice.

These extracts from the group dialogue highlight a culture of 'productive controversy', in contrast with a previous culture of the harmonious team. The real transformation is creating conditions where caring become possible rather than the individual work with patients and families that took place within an unsympathetic environment. Now a high level of mutual trust, acceptance, and support exist through the recognition of the emotional labour of practice. There is an overall feeling of 'being cared for'.

Conclusion

We have taken the lid off supervision and exposed some of the issues grounded in a research project that deliberately used line managers as supervisors who wanted to introduce supervision into their practices. In our blackest moments we feel that guided reflection will fail against the sharp edge of organisation, and the product model will become the norm. We feel this is predictable because organisations will implement supervision according to where they are coming from. The risk is that it will become another technology, rather than a way of being in the world. Perhaps the emphasis needs to be on reflective practice as an empowering and transformative process, and the question 'how can reflective practice best be guided?' needs to be asked.

Indeed reflection always begs the question, how can we create better worlds for ourselves and for the people we work with where our visions of caring and healing can be realised? Or in other words, how can we transform organisations from being primarily concerned with their own power interests into being primarily concerned with the interests of the people they exist to serve? One of the strongest images we have of this work is the power of the realisation and assertion of caring to change organisations. Fay (1987) described a critical social science as a process of enlightenment, empowerment, and emancipation from conditions that constrained people from achieving their best interests, oppressed by the power interests of others. Indeed this could be a description of nursing and nurses. This process, as Brendan's dialogues have illustrated, is a tough learning journey for both supervisors and practitioners, but through commitment, it is transformative.

References

Argyris, C. & Schön, D.A. (1989) *Theory in Practice: Increasing Professional Effectiveness*, 2nd edn. Jossey-Bass, London.

Blocher, D.H. (1983) Towards a cognitive developmental approach to counseling supervision. *The Counseling Psychologist*, **11**(1), 27–34.

Borders, L.D. & Leddick, G.R. (1987) *Handbook of Counseling Supervision*. The American Association for Counseling and Development, Virginia.

Dewey, J. (1936) *How We Think*. J.C. Heath, Boston.

Fay, B. (1987) *Critical Social Science*. Polity Press, Cambridge.

Foucault, M. (1979) *Discipline and Punish; The Birth of the Prison*. Vintage/Random House, New York.

Habermas, J. (1971) *Knowledge and Human Interests*. Beacon Press, Boston.

Hall, L. (1964) Nursing – what is it? *The Canadian Nurse*, **60**(2), 150–54.

Jarvis, P. (1992) Reflective practice and nursing. *Nurse Education Today*, 12, 174–81.

Johns, C.C. (1993) Professional supervision. *Journal of Nursing Management*, **1**(1), 9–18.

Johns, C.C. (1995) The value of reflective practice for nursing. *Journal of Clinical Nursing* 4, 23–30.

Johns, C.C. (1996) Visualising and realising caring in practice through guided reflection. *Journal of Advanced Nursing*, 24, 1135–43.

Johns, C.C. (1997) *Becoming an effective practitioner through guided reflection*. Unpublished PhD thesis. Open University, Milton Keynes.

Manthey, M. (1980) *The Practice of Primary Nursing*. Blackwell Science, Boston.

McCormack, B. & Hopkins, E. (1995) The development of clinical leadership through supported reflective practice. *Journal of Clinical Nursing*, 4, 161–8.

NHSME (1993) *Vision for the Future*. Department of Health, London.

Roberts, S.J. (1983) Oppressed group behaviour: implications for nursing. *Advances in Nursing Science*, **5**(4), 21–30.

Rogers, C. (1983) *Freedom to Learn for the 80s*. Charles E. Merrill Publishing Co., London & Ohio.

Schön, D.A. (1991) *The Reflective Practitioner: How Professionals Think in Action*, 2nd edn. Avebury, Aldershot.

UKCC (1996) *Guidelines for implementing clinical supervision*. United Kingdom Central Council for Nursing, Midwifery and Health Visiting, London.

Chapter 7
Illuminating the Transformative Potential of Guided Reflection

Christopher Johns

Introduction

The reflective practitioner is the creator of her world. By becoming sensitive to self within the context of everyday practice, she strives to be therapeutically available. This position assumes that reflection is always consciously motivated towards therapeutic intention. Within a human caring science such as nursing, therapeutic intention needs to be known in practice, rather than as a set of values or beliefs. Reflection-on-experience creates the opportunity for the practitioner to reflect on the meaning of caring beliefs and to expose, understand and actively work towards resolving the contradictions between caring beliefs and actual practice. Over time, the practitioner can look back at this experience and see self as a changed person, to see self reflexively, as transformed.

To achieve this requires what Fay (1987) describes as an *active stance* towards creating the conditions where the practitioner can be most therapeutically available. Fay's description of an active stance needs to be viewed within the context of a critical social science that intends to enlighten people as to the nature of the crisis within their lives, and on the basis of this enlightenment, to take action to emancipate self, empowered by this new understanding. In doing so the crisis and the suffering it causes are alleviated. The appropriateness of drawing on Fay's understanding of critical social science is evident within the way he conceptualises critical social science as, at once scientific, critical and practical.

Fay describes 'critical' as the 'sustained negative evaluation of the social order on the basis of explicit and rationally supported criteria' (p. 26). By 'practical' Fay means how practitioners were stimulated to act on the basis of new understandings to transform the conditions under which they worked towards the realisation of their best interests. This can only be the intention of reflection. The systematic recording of shared experience as dialogue within guided reflection sessions over time provides the basis for an understanding of the impact of guided reflection in enabling practitioners to realise desirable work as everyday practice, as a 'scientific' process. Whilst practitioners do not necessarily present 'in crisis', the intention within reflection is always to compare existing practice with beliefs and values, and consider the contradictions between beliefs and values and practice. Where no contradiction is manifest, the intention is then to consider the held beliefs and values and existing professional relationships for their appropriateness, within a wider understanding about the desirable nature of nursing – in other words to understand what desirable practice is and what it means to be effective in achieving it. What it means to be an 'active being' is conceptualised by Fay (1987) as best 'explicated in terms of four fundamental dispositions: intelligence, curiosity, reflectiveness, and wilfulness.' (p. 48) (Fig. 7.1).

Intelligence – The disposition to alter one's beliefs and ensuing behaviour on the basis of new information about the world.
Curiosity – The disposition to seek out information about one's environment in order to provide a fuller basis for one's assessments.
Reflectiveness – The disposition to evaluate one's own desires and beliefs on the basis of some such criterion as whether they are justified by the evidence, whether they are mutually consistent, whether they are in accord with some ideal, or whether they provide the greatest possible satisfaction, all in aid of answering the questions: what is the proper end of my life and thus what sort of person ought I to be?
Wilfulness – The disposition to be and to act on the basis of one's reflections.

Fig. 7.1 Fay's fundamental dispositions to being an 'active being'.

The extent to which the practitioner is inclined towards these four dispositions determines the extent to which the practitioner can transform herself in order to achieve desirable work. The 'evidence' is lived experience. 'Intelligence' and 'curiosity' are pre-requisite to reflection, while wilfulness is the commitment towards desirable work and the sense of empowerment necessary to act towards achieving this.

Contradiction

Fay's description of reflectiveness acknowledges the centrality of contradiction between beliefs and desires and the evidence of a lived life. Through reflection, these contradictions become visible along with the factors, both embodied within self and embedded within the environment, that contribute to the maintenance of these contradictions (Cox, *et al.* 1991). These authors focus action towards contradiction resolution that explicitly means transforming self:

'As we come to expose these self-imposed limitations, then the focus of our reflection shifts towards new action, towards the ways in which we might begin to reconstruct and act differently within our worlds.' (p. 387)

However, exposing these 'self-imposed limitations' may not necessarily be easy, and may require confrontation. Practitioners may feel more comfortable adhering to 'false beliefs' or what Lather (1986) labels as 'false consciousness' – 'the denial of how our common-sense ways of looking at the world are permeated with meanings that sustain our disempowerment' (p. 264).

However, this denial tends not to be conscious as in everyday life people take for granted the way things are. It is difficult to see beyond self, to see self as different. Indeed, the world may be a securer place adhering to the known and comfortable. Mezirow (1981) talks about 'disorienting dilemmas' and how the 'traumatic severity of the dis-orienting dilemma is clearly a factor in establishing the probability of a transformation' (p. 7). It is this sense of disorientation that brings the person to pay attention to the experience, although a more deliberative stance can be developed as the practitioner becomes increasingly sen-sitive to themselves in the context of what they are trying to achieve. The learning opportunity within reflection-on-experience is the attempt to resolve the contradictions between what the practitioner aims to achieve and how they actually practised within the specific experience. What the practitioner aims to achieve is never taken on face value but is itself open to scrutiny for its appropriateness and consequences.

Anäis' experience

The potential of guided reflection to bring about transformation is illu-strated through an experience shared by Anäis. She works as a Mac-millan nurse within a small team with whom I have been working for over two years in group guided reflection. We meet every 4 weeks for $1\frac{1}{2}$ hours. The group had initially approached me to facilitate their support group.

Anäis first shared this experience in session 29. The text is recon-structed from guided reflection dialogue recorded verbatim within the session. I encouraged Anäis to keep a reflective journal between sessions and to use the model of structured reflection (Johns 1995) in preparation for sharing within the group. Within the text, Clare is a colleague of Anäis. On this occasion Anäis recalled from memory.

> **Anäis:** He's a young lad, he's 27. He has had a liposarcoma surgically removed from his leg. This was diagnosed in 1994. Now he has secondaries in his spine, with symptoms of spinal cord compression. This has been treated with radiotherapy until he was mobile again. There was a 90% chance of short-term response but the chance is that it will be recurring. The hospital was anxious about him and hence they referred him to the district nurse. She contacted me and we arranged to make an initial joint visit. He had moved back home with his parents. His mother and father are very closed. On the day

of the visit I arrived slightly early. I knocked on the door but had no reply. They were in the garden and didn't hear me. I left. The district nurse arrived later and made the visit. She informed me that he didn't want Macmillan nurse involvement, that he was happy with her.

However, after 2 months she felt that she was getting nowhere with him – no communication. She felt the mother was blocking it on a social level. The district nurse asked me to become involved. She had suggested this to Simon, so I phoned him and suggested that he visit me at the clinic in the light of how difficult it had been for the district nurse at his home. He agreed with that. He first visited with his brother. It went all right and he agreed to visit again. But now after 7 sessions, I feel we are going round in circles with him. I don't know what to do next – it seems blocked.

Clare: Can you get him to say how he views the future?

Anäis: That's the issue, he doesn't see any future ... my sense of going around in circles. I can't seem to break through this.

I painted a picture of how I saw Simon: I have an image of a black cloud that obliterates his horizons.

Anäis: It's exactly like that.

CJ: Using visualisation with him may be useful. You could ask him to visualise where he is. What do you think he might say?

Anäis: It's difficult to say. It's difficult to envisage using this technique because I haven't used it before.

CJ: Use your imagination. Perhaps he would say he feels he is in a black pit where it is all dark and he cannot see in front of him. You might even suggest that image to him to begin to guide his visualisation. It's rather like painting a mental picture.

Anäis: But then what would I say?

I acknowledged Anäis' fear about using this technique. I suggested to her: If he says he can't see anything, then ask him to light a candle and ask him what he sees? You might actually light a candle for him. You can then ask him to explore the pit and see if there are any doors? Ask him what does he need to do to reach them, what does he hope to see if he goes through the doors? If he says he can't see any doors, suggest you can see one to his left. Just flow with it, use your imagination; there is no harm with it. Believe in yourself and your concern for Simon. I will see if I can find some literature on it. Perhaps you can look as well.

Anäis: Umm, it's interesting.

CJ: Have you tried any form of touch with him?

Anäis: I obtained money from Macmillan for him to have full body massage. He agreed to that, and said that it had helped him. It helped him feel relaxed but it has not helped him express his feelings.

CJ: How might he react if you gave him a hug?

Anäis: I couldn't do that!

CJ: Why not?

Anäis: I don't know how he might react to that. He is very shy, alone. He doesn't have a girlfriend.

CJ: Perhaps a hug might overwhelm him. You must use your judgement in knowing how to respond appropriately. However you also need to confront yourself – would you avoid touch because of your *own* discomfort? Touch can be a taboo.

In this context, I referred Anäis to the work of Jourard (1971), and noted

Lawler's study (1991) that suggested body work was largely invisible behind the metaphor of the 'screens'.

I continued: Do you shake his hand when you meet him?

Anäis: I do.

CJ: Perhaps hold his hand slightly longer, to express your concern for him and to let him know that he is not alone.

Anäis: Yes, I probably don't hold his hand any longer than I need to because I sense his discomfort, and my own discomfort.

CJ: What message would that give you, if it were you?

Anäis: Yes ... it would tell me you cared for me.

This was another visualisation of self, of putting self into the situation of receiving self's care. Clare asked if Simon had cried at all.

Anäis: No he hasn't. He has bottled all this up inside.

CJ: Perhaps something like touch could trigger his emotional release if you feel that appropriate at this time. Other ways of sharing his feelings might be through art, by asking him to draw a picture of himself right now. I noted a recent paper by Mayo (1996) that explored the use of art as enabling the expression of deep sub-conscious feelings, where feelings are expressed as pictorial metaphors.

I continued: Perhaps if you sense his discomfort with these types of inter- ventions you could express your thoughts with him – give him feedback that you perceive this, and help him talk about why he is uncomfortable with these. Similarly you could say to him something like, 'Simon, we have been working together now for seven sessions, let's review where we have reached and where we are going? You could say, 'I feel at a loss to know how best to help you', whilst acknowledging his feelings.

Anäis: I can understand that he can't concentrate. All he thinks about is what could happen to him. He says the right things to make me feel O.K. He makes me feel that I want to mother him.

CJ: You are suffering for him?

Anäis: He is frightened of dying, of being in pain, of being dependent. The relationships with his family – he can't talk to them. As he says, 'I come from a traditional Scottish family'.

Clare asked: Is he angry?

Anäis responded: He is not outwardly angry ... it's channelled inside him.

CJ: As represented by this black cloud, that's devouring him, obliterating him. I acknowledged Anäis' own sense of suffering for Simon. I recognised her strong need to to find a solution for Simon, to help him feel positive about his future, and how nurses often needed to do this as a consequence of their compassion. It was as if their compassion was a trap (Dickson 1982). I noted that many of Anäis' previous experiences had involved this sense of help- lessness in the face of distress with her consequent need to find a solution when that seemed so difficult – the need to feel useful, as a mother would for her child. Using transactional analysis (Stewart and Joines 1987) to frame this response pattern was helpful for Anäis to see herself as a nurturing mother to this helpless child, suffering, unable to help himself. This was an appropriate response at this time. Anäis represented a safe place. Anäis needed to recognise this need and her own response. As Anäis knew, there would come a time when Simon could move on. Our tactics had been aimed at helping Simon to move on, which required the expression of his angst, to make the connection between his present and his past, to acknowledge his loss and to acknowledge his future. Marris (1986) has noted that this temporal flow of connection is essential in dealing with loss.

I said to Anäis: Your work – to counter this need to fix-it for him. Think 'be there' for him. Perhaps you have to acknowledge that this is the intervention – he will recognise your concern and value your 'being there' for him. Perhaps at this time he cannot move forward ... you can't dictate this pace for him.

Anäis: I know you're right but it's so hard to see him suffering like this. It's such a shame.

Anäis had absorbed Simon's distress. She felt pity for him. While this is a natural human response it is not necessarily helpful, as it left her entangled in this emotional web that may compromise her ability to help him at this time. Levine (1986) offers a helpful view of compassion as being an opening of the self to the other. Levine contrasts with this 'pity', which is a reflection of the self's own concerns. I use the word compassion to reflect the mixture of empathy and concern, i.e. a knowing concern. It is the first manifestation of what 'therapeutic use of the self' means.

CJ: You know him quite well now. What were his interests before this?

Anäis: He has always been very interested in football. He had to give up playing that and lost his friends associated with that.

CJ: It might be useful to tune into what was positive in his life, his losses, even if that is all he talks about it – for example, how does he feels about Alan Shearer's transfer to Newcastle United. Hence to focus on 'what this event has meant to him' – rather than 'how does he see the future'.

These are reflective cues within the Burford NDU Model: Caring in Practice (Johns 1994), which I encouraged Anäis to use to frame her approach to patients and families.

Anäis: I did wonder if I was the best person to help Simon?

CJ: Are you?

Anäis: The fact that I feel I am going round in circles and feel frustrated suggests I may not be the best person. Perhaps he needs more specialist help?

CJ: Have you discussed this with his GP?

Anäis: I have. He responded by prescribing Simon some anti-depressants.

CJ: The medical model's limited response. Perhaps it would be an appropriate intervention to refer to other help; perhaps some sort of spiritual guidance may be helpful? We can link this back to getting Simon to reflect on your relationship and surfacing your sense of frustration with him. What options are there for referral?

Anäis and I explored these possibilities.

CJ: This is tough work for you. It highlights your own need for support.

Anäis: It has been hard. I know I take on board his feelings.

CJ: See how this unfolds when you next go in. We can revisit it next session.

In our next session Anäis said: I did the visualisation technique. I didn't have time to do any reading about visualisation. I was aware that I was going to see him next Tuesday. He came as planned and we went into the room where we normally meet. The environment of this room has now been improved, with more comfortable chairs – it is relaxing, warm, friendly.

One change was noticeable: he seemed so open, more talkative. He hadn't been like this before. I gave him that feedback and asked what had changed for him? He said that he had had four good weeks and felt more positive. I asked him what had happened. He said, 'I feel now I can actually start planning ahead'. He also said that he was reassured by what I had told him about spinal cord compression symptoms; I had informed him that he would get signs of this. He had feared that he would suddenly collapse. He felt that had actually helped, even though I had told him all this before! But perhaps he hadn't taken it in before. It went quiet. I'm not comfortable with long silences so I thought I would use visualisation. I said to him, 'Imagine you are in a dark room - what can you see?'

CJ: Did you ask him to close his eyes?

Anäis: No, but he didn't look at me. He was looking at the floor. It was amazing. He said, 'I see a door partly open. I've had this feeling of a black room in my dreams; its always unpleasant.' I said to him, 'Can you go beyond it, open it?' (Anäis said to me, 'I've never done this before') He said, 'I feel I can go through it because I can do my writing again'. Writing was one thing he used to do. He explained that that week he had written a letter to the *Daily Mirror* about how he had decided to go to the Disability Centre about work – it was on the top floor! He said it had made him laugh. He had been so sarcastic about this fact, and he won £25 as the star letter. It was really positive feedback for him. Writing is something he has always enjoyed. It was good he could use that experience so positively. I felt much more at ease than in the previous session with him. Is that why I could do it – use this technique?

He then started talking about his feelings of jealousy – about his friends and family – that they can go through life without questioning it. He talked in particular about his brother who had mocked him because he had a walking stick. He said, 'I didn't let them know they hurt me'. He said that he was very closed at home, and hid his emotions.

CJ: Perhaps that's his brother's way of coping with this – by being jokey?

Anäis: Yes, as Simon does with me. He blocks me with humour. I said to him, 'Where do we go from here?' He said, 'Am I going to benefit from it?' I replied, 'We have been going over old ground'. He said, 'I don't mind if you don't want to see me any more. Everybody else has done that.' He listed the physiotherapist, the hospital, the district nurse. He continued, 'But that's O.K.'.

I informed him that I was going on a break and would see him again in five weeks. I am also going on a course but I didn't tell him when. The course is six months. This relationship with him could go on for ever. I fear he is becoming dependent on me.

CJ: Why would you fear that?

Anäis thoughtfully: I don't know why, probably because I've got him to speak about things he's never spoken about to others before. I know why! He said, 'If I let go of you then something is going to happen to me'. He is frightened; he says everything's going to be all right but it isn't.'

Rachel interjected: Is that a problem?

CJ: See your relationship with him as a process unfolding over time. You had 7 sessions with him which left you feeling helpless and now this breakthrough ... perhaps the opposite is happening, perhaps he is beginning to take responsibility for his life but needs your support to do that. Perhaps it's your own concerns of feeling protective towards him that lead you to label him as dependent?

Anäis: I am anxious about being dependent on others, for example with the visualisation.

CJ: Perhaps it might help to see 'dependence' as a parallel process. You are anxious that he is dependent on you and you are anxious that you are dependent on others to support you. It is as if you do not feel in control. You are not omnipotent – you do not have all the answers. That is one reason you have supervision?

Anäis laughed: I couldn't hug him!

CJ: What about keeping him on whilst you do your course?

Anäis: I am anxious about closing with him when we meet next. He would find it hard for someone else to cover me during the 6 months.

CJ: You sound as if you are going to feel guilty.

Anäis: Yes, the responsibility is great. I don't know. The next 3 months I am definitely not around, but the second 3 months I will be on a community placement and could see him.

CJ: So that's one way of dealing with the problem – to tell him that?

Anäis: I don't know how he would take it.

CJ: Give him that decision to make.

Anäis: Yes – that would also encourage him to take responsibility.

CJ: I find this dependence interesting. If you look back over your relationship with Simon, his greatest need has been to find a safe place – where he can curl up. He has been dependent on you – that has been the therapeutic response. Developing the idea of visualisation, draw him a line on a large sheet of paper and mark the ends:

dependent ———————————— independent

Mark on the sheet where you think he has been on this line over the weeks.

Anäis excitedly responded: I could ask him to mark where he sees himself!

CJ: Yes, then ask him what this means for him.

Anäis: Something else we talked about – he has gone back to his Catholic religion. He wears his cross under his shirt. He says it's all inward, that he is doing it by himself. He hasn't shared it with his family.

CJ: That's interesting in the light of how we talked about his spiritual needs last session. Perhaps he might be encouraged to visit a priest?

Anäis: I could do that.

CJ: How do you feel now?

Anäis: I feel good about it now. I really do feel for him. I find that hard. I find it hard when he tells me he watches others playing football. He said, 'If only I could kick that ball'. You get more involved with some people than others.

CJ: That's where your own support is vital.

Commentary

I help practitioners to make sense of their learning through reflection, using the 'being available' template (Fig. 7.2). This template also offers a useful framework to reflect deeper on the transformative moment.

Being available to work with the patient and family in desirable ways is the core therapeutic activity of caring. The extent to which Anäis was available to work with Simon and his family is influenced by these dimensions. By looking back over time through the reflective lens offered by this template, Anäis can see the extent to which she became transformed, and the factors which both facilitated or limited this achievement.

The practitioner is available to work with the person (and family) to help them meet their health needs	Knowing what is desirable
	Concern
	Knowing the person
	Grasping, interpreting, envisaging what might be and responding with appropriate intervention
	Knowing and managing self
	Creating and sustaining the environment where being available is possible

Fig. 7.2 'Being available' template (Johns 1996)

Knowing what is desirable

Anäis strongly felt her work was centred in her relationships with individuals and with families from a unitary holistic perspective (Rogers 1986). From this perspective she sought to establish a level of involvement and intimacy within her relationship with Simon whereby she could be available for him to utilise her as part of his healing field.

Concern

Anäis' concern for Simon and her commitment to work strongly infused the dialogue. Simon mattered deeply to her. It is this concern which motivates her to confront her distress. Perhaps the key role of guidance is to infuse Anäis with the courage, knowledge and support necessary to confront the situation and take subsequent appropriate action – the balance of high challenge and high support. It is nurturing Fay's sense of wilfulness.

Knowing the patient

We can only nurse what the patient allows us to see (Hall 1964). Simon lived in his dark world in which Anäis stumbled and struggled to throw light on his darkest thoughts and feelings. Her frustration is a reflection of her failure to penetrate this dark world and know Simon. Reflection offered a light for Anäis to see Simon in a different way, to read his 'pattern' that rippled along the surface of how he presented to the world. By reading Simon's 'pattern', Anäis can come to understand the deeper meanings of this health event for him (Newman 1994, drawing on Bohm's theory of implicate order).

Responding with appropriate action

Anäis' story is infused with exploring appropriate ways of responding, and reflecting on their potential consequences. The practitioner's response within any clinical situation is a process of grasping, interpreting, envisaging what might be, and responding with appropriate action (Johns 1995). Anäis will intuitively feel what is best. It is not possible to predict the best intervention. Her most difficult learning is to learn to let go of a need to 'fix-it' for Simon and to learn that caring is a primarily a process of 'being there' rather than using a bag of tricks. Perhaps the most significant learning was knowing the right moment to take the appropriate action. By 'being there' Anäis can be ready for this moment rather than forcing the moment in her need to 'fix-it'. Anäis knew this, I just had to remind her. This knowledge had become blurred because she desperately wanted to help Simon and feel useful. She felt useless and helpless. We had often reflected-on this phenomena. Understanding this dynamic helped Anäis to check her own sense of failure and her consequent sense of frustration toward Simon.

That this letting go was hard for her to achieve reflects how such ways of responding to the world are embodied and not easily changed, even though we know rationally that there is a better way of doing things. The process of change is often slow. Hence guided reflection is always process focused rather than outcome focused, otherwise frustration may be increased in the face of failure. Noting what is best reflects the ethical dimensions within any experience. For example, should she confront Simon with his behaviour at this time? What would be the consequences of this? The story highlights the possibilities of working in new ways even though these may be uncomfortable to contemplate. The effective practitioner is always striving to increase her repertoire of interventions. Interventions such as visualisation are powerful healing therapies.

The dialogue illustrates how I introduced Anäis to relevant theory to inform her and help her make sense of her experience. Alternatively, I often encouraged Anäis to seek out relevant literature for herself. This was not intended to prescribe Anäis' response. By introducing theory at the appropriate moment, it is more likely that Anäis will read the theory and be able to relate it to her knowing in practice. In this way Anäis can contextualise theory and, depending on its relevance to the actual situation, she can assimilate and transcend the theory within her personal knowing towards constructed knowledge (See Chapter 5). It is only through reflection that practitioners can meaningfully apply theory and research within their everyday practice.

Knowing and managing self

Anäis desperately wanted Simon to reciprocate her offered level of involvement. Simon resisted this because he was wrapped up in his own inward looking world. His failure to reciprocate led to a breakdown in this relationship and Anäis' sense of crisis. Because of her concern for Simon and her sense of failure to help Simon, she suffered in the face of his distress.

Benner and Wrubel (1989) have noted that the extent to which things matter to us sets up what is possible, but also sets up what makes us vulnerable. Anäis could no longer respond therapeutically because she had become entangled in this web of uncontrolled feelings. The skill was for Anäis to tune into Simon, to literally get onto his wave length. Simon would then know her concern and she could remain involved as appropriate without absorbing Simon's distress and becoming anxious. I call this the 'caring dance' – the ability to synchronise self with other. The solution for Anäis is not to stop caring but to find new ways of coping in order to sustain caring.

Working with young dying patients is distressing. Numerous shared experiences give substance to this claim. Part of this coping is through understanding what is happening, part is acknowledging such feelings as human and valid. It is difficult work and yet it is vital work because such anxiety is energy draining. This understanding acknowledges that we live in a real world. It is important that Anäis acknowledges and accepts her limitations.

Through guided reflection Anäis can be helped to understand these dynamics and slowly chip away at her limitations. Just between two sessions, Anäis experimented with new ways of responding with good effect.

Creating the conditions where being available is possible

Anäis notes the uncertainty of having time to spend with Simon in the future within the context of other priorities. She feels the pressure of time, seeking results after seven sessions.

Anäis noted the significance of environment in creating a comfortable place where Simon can feel relaxed. As a Macmillan nurse Anäis manages her time and priorities, yet the service was under resourced in terms of staff, which put her time at a premium. This is perhaps the hardest work for practitioners – working in a world of depleted resources, often working within unresponsive and unsympathetic organisations, and working with other healthcare workers who are not mutually available to each other. Anäis was fortunate to work within a mutually supportive team. The effective practitioner becomes assertive, with a strong sense of powerful self, adept at political action to create an environment where being available becomes possible and practitioners such as Anäis can realise their therapeutic potential.

Guiding reflection as mutual growth

Facilitating Anäis' experience was a moving and intimate experience, to feel her compassion and distress for this young dying man. It nurtured the caring relationship between us in guided reflection. I was responding to Anäis in a way that paralleled her own approach to Simon. I had to know Anäis through her experience with Simon. My effort was to grasp the meaning this experience had for her, and based on this understanding to respond most appropriately. This suggests that I needed considerable knowledge and experience to draw on. However, whilst I am skilled at guiding reflection, my practical knowledge of using therapies such as guided imagery is limited. My response had been inspired by reading an account of a practitioner's use of guided imagery (Madrid 1990). Madrid's account concerned using guided imagery in working with a patient dying of AIDS. I felt that most significant was my ability to imagine what this experience was like for Simon, difficult as that is. Yet such empathy is central for understanding the other's experience. As the text illustrated, my imaging or empathy was spot on. As such, I learnt through this experience to respond more appropriately to practitioners such as Anäis within this profoundly moving experience.

Pursuing the idea of a parallel process between Anäis' relationship with Simon and my relationship with Anäis, the most difficult issues I confronted were to resist Anäis' need to 'fix-it' and to resist absorbing her distress. I had to help Anäis imagine 'dumping' her distress within the literal space between us and then seeing it for what it was. Just as practitioners like to feel useful, so do supervisors. But my skill was in being available for Anäis to use me as a resource, just as this was her key therapeutic role in working with Simon. Transformation is about the whole person, not merely the illness part of the person. The essence of transformation is to enable the other to make good decisions about their life based on understanding and a sense of freedom to act on these decisions (Newman 1994, drawing on Arthur Young's theory of evolutionary consciousness).

Conclusion

Anäis' work with Simon was unpredictable and presented as a crisis because normal ways of knowing and responding to the world were inadequate. The crisis was the learning opportunity accessible through reflection, enabling both Anäis and Simon to emerge with new insights that enabled more adequate responses. Simon, Anäis and myself are transformed within a process of expanding consciousness (Newman 1994) as we grow through the experience to fulfil our potential and destiny as human beings, even in suffering. The crisis was the transformative moment for us all to emerge at a higher level of human functioning congruent with desired ways of being (Newman 1994, drawing on Prigogine's theory of dissipative structures).

My thanks to Anäis, and to Margaret Newman for her work *Health as Expanding Consciousness* which provided me with a nursing theory with which to frame the process of guiding reflection as the means to facilitate transformation of self through experience. As a reflective practitioner, I have assimilated Newman's work within a wider theory of reflective caring, as outlined in Chapter 1.

References

Benner, P. & Wrubel, J. (1989) *The Primacy of Caring; Stress and Coping in Health and Illness.* Addison-Wesley Publishing, Menlo Park.

Cox, H., Hickson, P. & Taylor, B. (1991) Exploring reflection: knowing and constructing practice. In *Towards a Discipline of Nursing* (eds G. Gray & R. Pratt), pp. 373–90. Churchill Livingstone, Melbourne.

Dickson, A. (1982) *A Woman in Your Own Right.* Quartet Books, London.

Fay, B. (1987) *Critical Social Science.* Polity Press, Cambridge.

Hall, L. (1964) Nursing – what is it? *The Canadian Nurse*, **60**(2), 150–54.

Johns, C. (1994) Constructing the BNDU model. In *The Burford NDU Model: Caring in Practice* (ed. C. Johns). Blackwell Science, Oxford.

Johns, C. (1995) Framing learning through reflection within Carper's fundamental ways of knowing. *Journal of Advanced Nursing*, 22, 226–34.

Johns, C. (1996) Visualizing and realizing caring in practice through guided reflection. *Journal of Advanced Nursing*, 24, 1135–43.

Jourard, S. (1971) *The Transparent Self.* van Nostrand, Norwalk.

Lather, P. (1986) Research as praxis. *Harvard Educational Review*, **56**(3), 257–77.

Lawler, J. (1991) *Behind the Screens: Somology, and the Problems of the Body.* Churchill Livingstone, Melbourne.

Levine, S. (1986) *Who Dies? an Investigation of Conscious Living and Conscious Dying.* Gateway Books, Bath.

Madrid, M. (1990) The participating process of human field patterning in an acute-care environment. In *Visions of Rogers' Science-Based Nursing* (ed. E. Barrett). National League for Nursing, New York.

Marris, P. (1986) *Loss and Change*, revised edn. Routledge & Kegan Paul, London.

Mayo, S. (1996) Symbol, metaphor and story: the function of group art therapy in palliative care. *Palliative Medicine*, 10, 209–16.

Mezirow, J. (1981) A critical theory of adult learning and education. *Adult Education*, **32**(2), 3–24.

Newman, M. (1994) *Health as Expanded Consciousness*, 2nd edn. National league for Nursing, New York.

Rogers, M. (1986) Science of unitary human beings. In *Explorations on Martha Rogers' Science of Unitary Human Beings*, (ed. V. Malinski) p. 23. Appleton-Century-Crofts, Norwalk.

Stewart, I. & Joines, V. (1987) *TA Today: A New Introduction to Transactional Analysis.* Lifespace Publishing, Nottingham & Chapel Hill.

Chapter 8
Transforming Nursing Through Reflective Practice

Judy Lumby

Introduction

The focus of my work has been the transformative potential of reflection as a strategy or process. Situated as I am in a clinical chair within a hospital and area health service, I move between the boundaries of research, education and practice in a way which enables a merging, indeed a collapsing, of all three. Having experienced and authenticated the transforming nature of various reflective strategies within my doctoral and postdoctoral work, I have continued to use reflection with students in educational programmes and with registered nurses at the bedside. The sustained use of reflective strategies within research, however, is more problematic if proposals are submitted to Australian funding bodies. The hierarchy of credibility resists any invasion by so called 'new paradigm' research, particularly as research funds dwindle nationally. Nevertheless I am convinced of the possibilities which are realised when reflective strategies are used to uncover the knowledge embedded within practice in its many manifestations.

My major concern when we work within frameworks of reflection has been the way we take for granted that transformation has occurred. What do we mean when we speak of transforming nursing? Are we talking about changing the practitioners, the practice or the profession? My sense of transformation within a practice-based discipline is that unless it is manifested in the actions of individuals, it is not transformation but something else. My understanding of transformation in nursing, medicine or any other health related profession, is the shift which occurs when knowing 'about' becomes knowing 'the wise thing to do' and acting on that realisation. Wise actions are different from knowledgeable actions. Wise health care policies and practices integrate the empirical, the experiental and the ethical to ensure practice which considers what is wrong and what is possible to do for the best possible human outcome. Facts alone are not sufficient for wise decision-making in such a complex arena where the needs of sick individuals may change rapidly. Ironically, the contemporary world of health care increasingly demands instant action, routine responses, and outputs determined mainly by length of stay, thus silencing the more complex measures such as individuals' quality of life. To balance these imperatives and ideologies, my experience has been that practitioners require opportunities to critically appraise their world of work in ways which validate their paradoxical lives – paradoxical in terms of balancing individuals' beliefs, values and actions in a world dominated by bureaucratic beliefs, values and actions driven by economic considerations.

It is interesting that reflection 'in' and 'on' practice has been adopted so wholeheartedly by nurses in education internationally, within minimal critique. In Australia it may be explained by the fact that most nurses prior to 1985 could not undertake higher degrees in their own disciplines of nursing and so moved to education and the arts. The influence of charismatic characters such as the philosopher and educationalist John Dewey (1958) and the educational activist Paulo Freire (1972), was overpowering to a group who perceived themselves as an oppressed group within a system which denied them access to higher degrees of disciplinary rights. And both men were interested in the pedagogy of the oppressed. They spoke of reflection as a key to change for individuals and communities, while Freire lived his theory in positive ways for his Brazilian people existing under an extremely oppressive regime. His literacy programmes worked toward the process named *conscientizacao*, ultimately a move to critical action. Such an awareness, beginning with reflecting on their daily lives, led individuals to imagine and plan how they could take control of certain parts of their lives. Freire names this integration as distinct from adaptation, when individuals are still controlled by others within a semblance of autonomy. This process of emancipation cost Freire the freedom to live in his own country for many years, which in itself reinforced the power of his work.

Understanding 'experience'

While experience has been defined in multiple ways across disciplines and time, it is rarely discussed prior to implementing reflective processes. A universal meaning is assumed. But what constitutes an experience for first year undergraduate students may not be the same for final year students or experienced nurses. And individuals take note of different things within the same context. Some of this has to do with learning styles, but it also results from the social and historical background of the individual. Without defining or at least discussing the parameters of an experience within a particular programme, students are disadvantaged and teachers confused.

John Dewey in his early work emphasised the nature of experience as a dialectic with the world, rather than an isolated, individualistic and irrational concept portrayed in scientific discourse. A recent experience with a research proposal of my own best illustrates the latter. A medical reviewer wrote that 'interviewing patients about their experiences will not get to the truth of the matter', the matter in this case being the experience of receiving a diagnosis of and undergoing surgery for colorectal cancer. The explicit message appears to be that patients cannot be trusted to recall their experience or to make any sense of it, while the implicit message is that knowledge and truth can only be found through an 'objective' observer (Polanyi 1958). The extensive philosophical critique of mind/body, nature/culture and theory/practice dualisms reveals the assumptions upon which research has been and is still evaluated in terms of what is valid and rigorous and therefore scientific. Reflection as a research tool or method continues to be perceived as questionable as far as issues of validity, reliability and generalisation are concerned, often forcing nurses to abandon such strategies or to manipulate them in a way which ensures loss of integrity.

Despite these barriers many nurses continue to be convinced of the power of using reflective strategies in education and scholarly inquiry. The explosion of texts addressing reflection and reflective practice perhaps best illustrates a frustration with traditional methods of inquiry, particularly inquiry into practice. For this reason teachers and nurses have been particularly interested in adopting reflective processes, either to uncover the complexities of the clinical world or the classroom or to empower practitioners in either setting, to utilise the invisible and often undervalued knowledge embedded in their practice. The way in which reflection has been embraced by practice-based disciplines also illustrates a belief in the multiple ways in which knowledge manifests itself. In particular, it emphasises the importance of theorising about the knowledge grounded in practice, which is often invisible to the untrained observer. Reflective processes are one way of beginning the process of theorising which is not linear but a reasoning dialectic between knowing and doing (Sartre 1968). This dialectic also captures many forms of knowledge, challenging the traditional privilege of technical (say, scientific) knowledge over other forms such as practical and emancipatory (Habermas 1974).

Layers of reflection

A major assumption in much of the literature on reflective processes is that they are inherently transformative. My experience with educational programmes which make this claim has reinforced the need for attention to the reflective strategies and methods of evaluation. There is often little evidence or evaluation of whether students have moved through to levels of critical reflection which may then claim to be transformative. My own doctoral work illustrates the complexity and layering of transformative processes, and Smith and Hatton's (1993) research over three years reinforces this. This research was initiated to challenge some of the assumptions inherent in the literature on reflective practice and to evaluate strategies to facilitate reflective practice within a Bachelor of Education degree at The University of Sydney. The outcomes of the research demonstrated that 60–70% of students reflected only at a descriptive level. This level of reflection involves describing events and actions and occasionally justifying an action.

The move to a level of critical reflection requires much more in terms of process and facilitation, since it is here that transformation links reflection and revisioning. When we revision, we 'see again', revising previous assumptions and identifying possibilities never imagined. We become aware of the multiple perspectives of events and actions, the historical and socio-political contexts in which they are located. This is when the known becomes part of the knower, the observed becomes part of the observer and the interpreted becomes the interpreter (Lumby 1992). In this way individuals are able to move to levels of critical understanding rarely reached through the written word alone, although combined with oral telling, the written word can be a powerful and simultaneous act of knowing and doing, leading to a transformed and collective wisdom. Wheeler and Chinn's (1992) work with women across cultures is illustrative of this, as is the work of indigenous groups who pass their collective wisdom across generations through story-telling, acting, singing and dancing.

The reflective journey

Reflective practice has been part of my life as a nurse, a woman and a mum forever. It was not a new concept when I came across it during my studies in education; it was in me so I knew it immediately. The most difficult step was utilising it within my doctoral work, which involved journeying with one woman as she experienced a life-threatening illness in the form of biliary cirrhosis and ultimately a liver transplant. This journey was one I was invited into just as nurses are invited into journeys with patients every day. Maree, a distant colleague whom I had only met once, rang me to ask for help, although that is not what she said. But we know cries for help. They are not explicit; they are bound up in language like 'I feel stunned!', followed by a description of a professional encounter often poorly handled. Maree reminded me of where we had met and then said, 'I have just been told to go out and live until I die. How can you live knowing you are going to die?' I was to hear this impossible-to-answer question again and again over the next six years, not only from Maree but from others who had experienced the same paradoxical dialogue. And so began this journey of critical reflection, with two women telling stories to each other and making meaning of their journey together and individually. Ultimately this transformed our lives forever as women, nurses, daughters and mothers. For Maree her experience was validated through a process of shared sustained reflection and critical inquiry. As she tells us:

'The search has validated the significance of the experience for me. It has turned it from just an operative procedure to save my life into an experience which has been life changing, where I had to look and acknowledge why there had to be life changing attitudes. I look at myself compared to 5 years ago and I am just so different. I think all the experiences that I have been through have certainly contributed to that, but I think the biggest thing is that I have had to look at it all and learn to understand ... that I have learned to understand that it has meaning and value.' (Lumby 1992, p. 74)

And it was through reflective processes that Maree was led to look at it and to discover the meaning and value in her experiences. The processes used in this study were carefully chosen for their well validated transformative qualities. These included story telling and incidental and sustained reflective inquiry. Shulamit Reinharz, a feminist social scientist, informed some of this work through her text on experiential analysis (Reinharz 1979). By experiential she means a spiral process of interactivity involving continual reflection, analysis and synthesis individually and collaboratively. But even using such processes I needed to take several more steps and try out a variety of strategies before I was sure we were moving to a level of critical awareness where entrenched beliefs, values and practices were questioned. Even when this questioning began, it did not mean that transformation was a natural outcome. After all, we question things daily but this does not necessarily lead to a transformation of our lives in any way. My interest lay within the space between critical reflection and revisioning. It is here that transformation occurs. Revisioning is when one views the old with new eyes, seeing possibilities not previously imagined. When this happens there has been a transformation.

The multi-layering of meaning-making which I employed was to ensure a rich text, along with an authentication of the narrative. For two women intimately involved over two years in the experiences, it also meant that we were able to reach a level of critical awareness only possible when relationships are trusting and safe. Feminist and other writers confirmed my experiences of story telling as therapeutic (Gilligan, 1982; Brody, 1987; Raymond, 1986), while other writers had begun to explore the so called 'new' paradigms of research, confirming my belief that research has a wider focus than determining cause and effect. The process of research in and of itself can be transforming for both the researcher and those involved as participants – the co-researchers. In this way I understand it as contributing to a wise society, not merely a knowledgeable one.

My initial dilemma was how do I work with a dying woman in a way which not only does not harm but actually makes her journey more bearable. At the beginning, transplantation was not an option so we began the study as one in which we journeyed through her dying together. Six months into the study she was offered a liver transplant and we continued the study for another 18 months until she felt able to remove herself and 'get on with her new life'. The form of the study, explained briefly below, revealed itself only in the final stages, as most transformative experiences do if we are reflective in intent.

Phase 1 – searching for meaning

This phase involved Maree and I taping our 'incidental reflections'. My tapes consisted of responses to her almost nightly, often despairing telephone conversations. These tapes were mainly from the perspective of a mother since we both had three daughters and she was contemplating how to tell hers of her impending death. Her tapes were recorded at night as she lay in bed and spoke to me on tape about her innermost fears and her hopes for the future. We then had what I have called 'joint conversations', when I took Maree out to a garden or to a cafe for a chat, as women do. The only difference was that we had a tape recorder between us on which we used to record our conversations. Later we exchanged our individual tapes to create 'shared reflections'. Nine months into the taping, when she was very debilitated and closely contemplating death, Maree received an organ and underwent her liver transplant. We continued to tape our conversations until she was wheeled into the operating theatre, and later during my daily visits. Following her discharge I interviewed those people in Maree's life whom she nominated as influential. These were her three daughters, whom I interviewed separately, and her parents who insisted on being interviewed together.

Phase 2 – making meaning

This phase was the most emotionally difficult stage of the study since it was here that I introduced the critical phase so necessary for reflection to be transforming. 'Critical' in this study is used in the sense of artistic criticism. With art criticism, those involved engage in a socio-political interaction in which a work of art is judged or evaluated. Because it is important to try to understand the individual artist's reality (if this is ever possible), there is a certain empathy which is applied, just as in nursing where we try to understand the meaning of another's experience. So it was with us as we developed a process which I named critical conversations. This was the critical point of transformation for us both and could only have happened through the intensity of our work together over a sustained period. Our stories on tape informed us of the stories and biographies we had shared and so we continued to listen to each of these in chronological order. When we needed to critically appraise or question what we had recorded over time, we stopped the tape and recorded our dialogue on the matter at hand. The result was twelve critical tapes which held the essence of our transformative work, although ultimately transformation can only be evaluated in practice by actions.

Phase 3 – transforming meaning

The third phase was the time in which our journey began to unfold. We needed to know what had happened over that time. How did we make sense of it? What did it mean for the future of nursing, for others undergoing such experiences and for ourselves as women, daughters, mothers and nurses? Was it just a two year chat between two women as a medical colleague had suggested? Analysing the final critical tapes was extremely complex. They were the distilled essence of the two years. How to reflect the drama, the agony, the joy, the transformation through the text of a doctorate? Because of the feminist nature of the research, I began this phase by writing my narrative to Maree in which I shared my experiential understanding of the last two years. She replied with her narrative which then became our narrative. I began with this step because I rejected the idea of pulling our story apart into tidy boxes called themes, which seemed to destroy the authenticity of the study. Nevertheless, in order to portray some of the major dilemmas faced by Maree during her journey towards death, I did identify major themes which Maree then authenticated prior to their inclusion in the text.

Phase 4 – sharing our meaning

Phase 4 was the final stage. This ultimately was the climax of critical reflection, when theory and practice become one and could not be separated. This was praxis. We became the experience and our lives had been transformed forever. Margie Martin (1991) explains our experience exactly in her work on transformation metaphors, which is part of her doctoral work.

> 'The challenge of developing a methodology of practice has been to realise that the way I order my nursing knowledge per se is not in theories or in philosophy but within consciousness. Reflecting this statement back to myself led me to understand that a theory cannot heal; a theory is useful when it is useful. You cannot live your life through a theory.' (Martin 1991, p. 4)

> 'I discovered praxis to be the art of aligning theory and practice within consciousness. This reset my practice from a straight line into an opening curve.' (Martin 1991, p. 4)

This opening curve led Maree to take some life changing actions. She left an abusive marriage and six years later is alive in a way she never dreamed possible, living on a farm on the top of a mountain, symbolic of the mountain she and I climbed together. Here she has transformed the earth into a magnificent garden and is amazed daily by new growth.

Group reflection through shared stories

This doctoral work was followed by a two year study also informed by critical feminist thought. This later study involved eight members of a liver transplant support group, and once more story telling was used but within a focus group process. Reflection in this study was manifest through the synergy which is the strength of focus groups. As each member told their story of the monthly focus, such as being handed a diagnosis of death, this would trigger memories and stories for others in the group. The end result was the passing on of individual stories and the weaving of a collective story. Individuals in the group commented on the importance of the group process in enabling them to share their innermost stories. Despite the group having been formed for some time before the study, the stories shared in the focus groups had not been shared before. Somehow the framework of identifying a monthly focus and the pattern of circling the stories rather than using cross dialogue was releasing for the members. This is similar to Margie Martin's use of refracted rather than reflected images. As individual members storied about an experience during their illness and transplant, other members of the group were able to see an image refracted from the energy field of the story teller and to align with this image. While individuals in the group were identified in the statistics of the National Liver Transplant Unit as 'survivors', several were not surviving in personal and professional terms. Reflecting on such issues enabled them to see options not previously visible.

The power of story telling as a transforming process has informed much of my work since my doctorate. I have utilised it in education as well as research and several of my doctoral students are using it in their work. One has moved to Frigga Haug's memory work which is story telling used in areas of extreme sensitivity and trauma, such as a study of relinquishing mothers. Story telling as method has received increasing publicity in the research and nursing literature in the last few years (Reason & Hawkins 1988; Sandelowski 1991; Ayres & Pointer 1996). The attractiveness to nurses is the fact that stories are part of their practice. They are told stories every day, sometimes stories which have never been shared before. And they use such stories to inform the way in which they craft their practice. Because of this they understand only too well the therapeutic nature of story telling.

Mishler (1979) tells us that each story is embedded in and inextricable from its context. The researcher as interpreter of the story must therefore be sensitive to the way in which meaning is constructed from the narrated text. Ayres and Pointer speak of the fact that 'interpretation begins not with stories told aloud to the interviewer but with the transcript of story as received by the researcher' (Ayres & Pointer 1996, p. 164). The interview as transcribed becomes like a script. This assumes a very different story telling methodology from the one I have used and which is espoused in the feminist literature. It was for such reasons that I chose to work with Maree as a co-researcher, and to make, or interpret the meaning of, our stories together, rather than be the interpreter. It is also the reason for including Maree in the final drafts of the thesis, to avoid inauthentic representation of her story. We overcame the notion of the transcribed interview as a text by introducing our stage of critical conversations where we collaboratively made meaning of (interpreted) our stories, thus creating our own text of transformation.

Another venture in story telling has been that in which I attempted to capture the stories of care which are buried in the walls of hospitals. This occurred within a graduate programme, involving specialist nurses working in critical care units. The unit of study was about models of care within the health care system. Knowing that the knowers of such models were already there in the classroom, I chose to tap into such expertise by the use of stories of care over time. I chose story telling as the method because of the traditional models experienced by these students. In their previous studies, particularly in intensive care, they had been educated through the use of case studies. When I asked them to write about their nursing care I was given texts which I viewed as medical care. They were the traditional case studies produced and eulogised by doctors at scientific meetings, which begin with presenting symptoms and move through differential diagnosis, measurements, testing and then definitive diagnosis, treatment and so on. Nurses have followed this way of thinking because many have been taught by doctors, while nursing was not identified as valid knowledge.

But case studies, while useful, deny the person in the patient, which is the focus of nursing care. Case studies are analytical reports only, avoiding the ethical, the intimate and the social and cultural context of the person whose future is being planned. Because of this long history of the use of case studies as a mode of learning, the introduction of new ways of learning and thinking about thinking, requires a sensitive approach. In addition, story telling is identified as not really about learning and this adds to the initial concern expressed by students, particularly those coming from areas where complex technology is the central focus.

So it was that I spent a preparatory period at the beginning of the graduate course speaking of ways of knowing prior to introducing the idea of story telling as a method for making meaning. After several weeks, when the group appeared to be more receptive and even quite interested, we began our group story telling with the understanding that if the group believed that it was not appropriate, they had the right to ask for it to be changed. Every evening that we met we began the session with twenty minutes devoted to stories of care from two students in the group. There were no guidelines for the type of story or the context. The only criteria was that the story had to be from practice in which the student was involved in some way. The stories were extraordinary, and most involved ethical dilemmas. Many were sad and the story tellers often cried tears they had saved for years. Michael White (cited Kamsler

1990) identifies the therapeutic nature of story telling in his work with abused women. He identifies this as the re-authoring of the dominant story by the woman whose story has usually been told and authored by others. White speaks of the story teller as 'generating news of difference which makes a difference' (cited Kamsler 1990, p. 22).

Once more, with the student group as the focus, I recognised the refracted energy within the group which began a domino effect of remembering similar events. There was more similarity than difference in the stories despite a variety of contexts and people. Following each student story, the group were involved in a dialogue which was both supportive and critical in intent. Each week the tapes were transcribed and handed back to the authors for authentication. This in itself was quite a powerful process, as it had been for Maree during our doctoral work. Many students were overwhelmed with the way in which their story came to life in the written text. They commented on how powerful the process had been for them. Solfgang Iser and Frank Kermode (cited in Ayres & Pointer 1996, p. 164) suggest that the mere reading of a text triggers the interpretive process anyway, and I would add from experience that the mere listening to a story also triggers that process. Iser speaks of the artistic and aesthetic poles of the text which intersect to become the virtual text. And because each reading becomes another re-interpretation, meaning construction is never finalised.

Concept mapping

At the end of the stories I faced my previous dilemma. Narrative data certainly presents a methodological paradox (Ayres & Pointer 1996). How to make sense of these stories in a way which does not destroy the meaning of the whole yet enables students to use the stories to inform their practice? How to ensure the critical reflection which occurs over sustained periods in practice? After much discussion with the students involving story telling, the theories surrounding it and the practicalities of utilising story telling as a process of learning, I decided to work with concept mapping to develop a model of care which represented that group of nurses and their care. We also agreed to write a monograph using certain stories. For all the students this was their publication and they would also have their shared model of care which they could take with them to re-form their practice. Most spoke of the new level of critical awareness that the stories had raised for them. They felt challenged to question many of the taken-for-granted practices and hierarchical models of care within their world of work. We mapped their world of care through their stories, phrasing their concepts in the everyday language of health and illness care. The map became their collaborative model of care, which several have reminded me of years later.

Finally I would like to share one more experience I have had utilising reflection as a method of transforming practice. To achieve this I used mapping as a group exercise in a graduate diploma in critical care nursing. The unit of study was one which I had developed to raise awareness of the political, social, historical and environmental world in which specialised nurses worked. The unit was divided into these four worlds of the nurse, but prior to making this division I requested that the 50 students broke into six groups and mapped their world of work reflecting both the macro and micro world in which they worked. There were no guidelines for the maps, which at first they found disconcerting. Ultimately however they enjoyed the freedom to create their own interpretation of cartography. Each group then shared their map with the larger group.

The outcome was six maps of the world of the nurse. While each map was different in its presentation, in every one the nurse was graphically displayed in the centre of what appeared to be a centrifuge surrounded by a world of chaotic demands. The maps were powerful in their presentation of feelings and perceptions, revealing many of the fears and concerns within the groups. As the co-ordinator, I felt a sense of urgency to address some of the issues raised by the maps and to find ways of moving forward through planning strategies. Along with the larger group I then planned the remaining sessions of study to address some of the issues raised by the maps and to introduce constructive ways of overcoming the sense of powerlessness displayed by the design of the map. This mapping exercise proved to be a very powerful method for encouraging incidental and sustained individual and group reflection. Because it addressed the world of work, the map became a visible tool for 'dialogue and dialectic development' (Reason & Hawkins 1988, p. 84). This involves a meeting of the paths of explanation (denotative thinking) and expression (connotative thinking), so that the two methodologies can intersect and individuals can move across the two, thus entering the space between. This space is often one in which the participant can find a way of understanding and working which is different from the previous one in which they feel uncomfortable or alienated. I believe that many nurses work naturally in this space between the scientific and artistic worlds. Others may need to find the space.

Conclusion

Mapping and story telling are just two methods or processes which I have found particularly helpful and exciting to use with a group or with individuals. They are transformative because they assist individuals to move through the levels of reflection identified by Smith and Hatton (1993), which are descriptive, dialogic and critical. The descriptive level is often the level that students reach when writing reflective diaries, but it is only useful if students are also asked to provide some reasoning for actions taken. Dialogic reflection offers a stepping back from the actions or events. This enables a different level of discourse either with self or others and was reflected in the group dialogue after the student story telling and my doctoral work with Maree. The third level of reflection described by Smith and Hatton is critical reflection, in which there is an awareness that events and actions are located in and explicable by reference to multiple perspectives. Exploring political and social influences and contexts assists this awareness, which was experienced in the classes where mapping was used and ultimately through the use of critical conversation in my doctoral work. It was at this level that transformation of meaning occurred for Maree, myself as researcher and woman, and for both groups of students. Transformation also occurred personally as the processes used enabled individuals to see themselves in new ways, and to recognise the value of their work as nurses and the value of themselves as individuals.

References

Ayres, L. & Pointer, S. (1996) Virtual Text and the Growth of Meaning in Qualitative Analysis. *Research in Nursing and Health*, 19, 163–9.

Brody, H. (1987) *Stories of Sickness*. Yale University Press, New Haven.

Dewey, J. (1958) *Theory and Nature*. Dover Publications Inc., New York.

Freire, p. (1972) *Cultural Action for Freedom*. Penguin, Harmondsworth.

Gilligan, C. (1982) *In a Different Voice: Psychological Theory and Women's Development*. Harvard University Press, Massachusetts.

Habermas, J. (1974) *Theory and Practice*. Heinemann, London.

Kamsler, A. (1990) Her-Story in the making: therapy with women who were sexually abused in childhood. *Ideas for Therapy with Sexual Abuse* (eds M. Durrant & C. White), pp. 9–37.

Lumby, J. (1992) *Making meaning from a women's experience of illness; the emergence of a feminist method for nursing*. Doctoral thesis. Deakin University Library, Geelong, Victoria, Australia.

Martin, M. (1991) *Trans-form-ation metaphors; a critical action study of life forms in life challenging situations*. Science, Reflexivity and Nursing Care; Exploring the Dialectic, Australian National Nursing Conference.

Mishler, E.G. (1979) Meaning in Context: Is there any other kind? *Harvard Educational* Review. 49, 1–19.

Polanyi, M. (1958) *Personal Knowledge; Towards a Post Critical Philosophy*. Routledge and Kegan Paul, London.

Raymond, J. (1986) *A Passion for Friends; Towards a Philosophy of Female Affection*. Beacon Press, London.

Reason, P. & Hawkins, P. (1988) Story telling as inquiry. In *Human Inquiry in Action; Developments in New Paradigm Research* (ed. P. Reason) pp. 79–102. Sage Publications, London.

Reinharz, S. (1979) *On Becoming a Social Scientist: From Survey Research and Participant Observation to Experiential Analysis*. Jossey-Bass, San Francisco.

Sandelowski, M. (1991) Telling stories: narrative approaches in qualitative research. *Image*, 23, 161–6.

Satre, J.P. (1968) *Search for a Method*. (trans. by H. Barnes) Vintage Books, New York.

Smith, D. & Hatton, N. (1993) *Critical reflection on action in professional education*.

5th National Practicum Conference, February 1993. Macquarie University, Sydney.

Wheeler, C. & Chinn, P. (1992) *Peace and Power; A Handbook of Feminist Process* (3rd edn.) National League for Nursing, New York.

Chapter 9

Exploration of the Empowering Potential of Clinical Supervision, Reflection and Action Research

Carolyn Moore and Julia Carter

Introduction

The nursing process emanated from, and was reflective of, the positivist tradition which no longer dominates the nursing domain. But in spite of growing support for a movement away from the scientific objectification of nursing, nurses continue to be educated and to plan care through the systematic approach of problem solving. The literature supports the view that nursing has developed beyond the restrictions of an approach which threatens the art and creativity of therapeutic nursing (McHugh 1986; Benner & Tanner 1987).

We aim to demonstrate the way in which reflective practice can be a powerful tool in enabling nurses to begin to challenge established practice. The processes of action research, clinical supervision and reflective practice were brought together in an attempt to raise the collective consciousness of one group of practitioners. While the initial challenge was focused on changing the way in which care was planned and enabling patients to become more involved in their care, the raised awareness which ensued can be seen to have impacted upon the nurses 'way of being'. As individuals and as a group, the nurses in the study area became empowered to challenge not only themselves and their interactions with patients, but also some of the organisational constraints which impacted on their practice.

The next section of this chapter offers the reader some insight into the clinical area chosen for the project and gives not only a working definition of reflection but also some justification as to why it was viewed as crucial to the process of change. Further, a rationale is given for the adoption of action research as the most appropriate methodology to explore the change in practice. The difficulties associated with patient participation as a concept, and the way in which care planning worked in practice, are outlined in the following section of this chapter – 'What was the intended change?'. Here, both the practice concerns around the issue and concerns emanating from a review of the literature are highlighted, and a brief account of the tools of change are identified. In the following sections, 'The change process' and 'Recognition of change', a résumé is given of the action steps taken throughout the project and the methods I adopted in order to establish that a change in practice was happening. The section 'The change' offers a summary and discussion of what happened throughout the process as it was experienced by the participants, and utilises information arising from data collection and Julia's personal reflections. Finally, there is a presentation of some of the perceived limitations within the project.

The project took place over a relatively short period, and we do not claim to have changed our world. Our account outlines the beginnings of a process which impacted enough on the nurses working in the area for them to continue to strive for things to be different. The emphasis of this chapter is to explore the impact of reflection to bring about a change in clinical practice. This change is illustrated with the reflections of Julia, a staff nurse and participant in the project.

Background

Working as a practice development nurse, I was able to work closely with the staff and patients of ward six, a medical ward. The ward cared for a predominantly elderly population and was typical of many in relation to staffing levels and resources.

I chose an action research approach because of its potential to both manage the development of clinical practice and to monitor both the processes and outcomes (Luker 1992). The participants, the nurses on the ward, were seen as major stakeholders in the process (Koch 1994), implementing the change and participating in its evaluation. In this way there was a 'coming together' of the researcher and participants in seeking knowledge grounded in practice:

'Consciousness arises out of and is shaped by practice, and in turn is judged in and by practice.' (Mathews 1980, cited in Carr & Kemmis 1986)

Whilst it is true to say that the area of concern chosen was a reflection of a problematic issue for the nurses on ward six, the initial impetus for change was driven by my agenda. Holter and Schwartz-Barcott (1993) identify the 'enhancement approach' to action research, to raise the collective consciousness of practitioners by making fundamental problems explicit. This approach also aims to close the gap between actual problems encountered by professionals in a defined setting and the theory which is used to explain and resolve them. The emphasis is centred around bringing to the surface underlying value systems and was seen to be of crucial importance to the proposed change.

Ten qualified staff were already involved in the Department of Health project (Butterworth *et al.* 1996) exploring the impact of clinical supervision. Nurses were, for the first time, being asked to reflect on their practice and as a result, reflective skills were starting to develop. Whilst clinical supervision was not a planned part of the study, the fact that the nurses were involved in it influenced the decision to use this particular clinical area. With hindsight, it was crucial to its success.

I considered reflection fundamental in any attempt to challenge the received view of knowledge that nurses held at a practice level. Reflection on action was encouraged with the intention of revealing the process of, and exploring the multi-faceted nature of, change. The aim of utilising reflection was not primarily intended to facilitate learning through experience, but to gain insight into nurses' experiences to enable an understanding of how these experiences influenced the change process and to reveal factors which affected the process. All of the qualified nurses on the ward were asked to keep a reflective journal at the outset of the project, and at the end a volunteer sample submitted their journals for analysis. After a review of the theoretical approaches to reflection, I adopted the definition by Boyd and Fales (1983):

> 'The process of internally examining and exploring an issue of concern triggered by an experience, which creates and clarifies meaning in terms of self, and which results in a changed perspective.'

Whilst a little simplistic and narrow in definitive terms, it offered a starting point which enabled the participants to begin to explore how the issues coming to light matched, or otherwise, their personal values. At the time of the project's initiation, we were all starting out on the road of discovery and were not able to anticipate the impact and meaning that reflection would have.

What was the intended change?

The problem

My passionate belief in the potential of care planning as a tool which enabled the individualisation of care was being consistently challenged in the practice arena. The use of a computerised care planning system was lamented by practitioners who felt that their creativity was stifled. Care planning had become just another encroachment on the delivery of care, a time consuming task to be completed with little or no obvious benefit to the patient or to practitioners. Management were asking questions about the utility of care planning in terms of 'patient outcomes'. The potential was great for yet another 'off the shelf' package to be imposed on nursing.

If care planning was of value and more than 'record keeping' – i.e. it could offer a vehicle through which patient care could be individualised to meet the unique needs of patients – there was an urgent need for nurses themselves to take control and to determine a system of care planning which would work for the patient and for the nurse. An analysis of the literature surrounding the nursing process revealed a general and growing trend of dissatisfaction and negativity associated with its use. The criticism was wide ranging, from a general dissatisfaction (Palmer 1988; Taylor-Gwozdz & Del-Tongo Armanasco 1992) and a recognition that the nursing process was neither meeting its assumed aims (Henderson 1982; Davis *et al.* 1994), nor empirically proven to improve patient care (Sovie 1988; Ford & Walsh 1994), to the suggestion (now gathering momentum) that the nursing process was holding back the 'expert' abilities and skills of many practising nurses (Henderson 1982; McHugh 1986; Fonteyn & Cooper 1994). If the nursing process was to survive, there was clearly a need for urgent and methodologically mature research into the value of its use to patients.

Alternatively, Shea (1986) had questioned the feasibility of one system – the nursing process – in meeting the multiple aims attributed to it. It was clear that the complex needs of the patient and the unique skills of the nurse must in some way be documented. Some of the available alternatives to traditional care planning, for example, collaborative care planning and care pathways, were considered by the author and by the ward nurses to perpetuate the view of the patient as passive recipient and to have no greater demonstrable benefits than the nursing process. Thus, the second perhaps more ambitious aim was to increase the level of patient participation in the decision-making process.

Patient participation was seen as implicit and inseparable from the concept of individuality reflected within the infrastructures of nursing. However, whilst participation was viewed as inherent within concepts such as primary nursing and the nursing process, it was often assumed; the empirical evidence that practice matched the theoretical assumptions was lacking (Trnobranski 1994). Further, controversy exists over the notion of participation, and questions were being asked about its value; did patients either desire or benefit from greater involvement?

The tools

The traditional approach of the nursing process was challenged and the problem solving approach to care planning abandoned. A care planning system was introduced which aimed to re-focus the core of care planning to the patient. This was built on the concept of mutual goal setting, something which had been utilised elsewhere with some documented success in terms of staff satisfaction and improved patient outcomes (CURN Project 1982). A care planning system built on the concept of mutual goal setting provided a starting point for planning and documenting care. However, we needed an adequate framework for guiding the way the practitioner assessed and responded to patients in desirable ways.

The activities of living model which had previously underpinned the delivery of care was viewed as limiting; if we were to truly establish the concerns of patients, it could not be assumed that these would be centred around the predefined framework given in such a model. The Burford NDU Model, Caring in Practice (Johns 1994) (Fig. 19.1) offered a

---

What information do I need to be able to nurse this patient?

Cue questions:

- Who is this person?
- What health event brings them into hospital?
- How must this person be feeling?
- How has this event affected their usual life patterns and roles?
- How does this person make me feel?
- How can I help this person?
- What is important for this person to make their stay in hospital comfortable?
- What support does this person have in life?
- How do they view the future for themselves and others?

Fig. 9.1   Burford NDU Model: Caring in Practice (Johns 1994)

potential assessment tool grounded in holistic belief, which would hopefully enable the nurse to begin to view the patient in more holistic ways as desired. The Burford NDU model is itself a model of reflection, using the framework of reflective cues to 'tune' practitioner into the unit's philosophy for practice, within each clinical moment. The model explicitly acknowledges the caring moment as a simultaneous process of assessing what is, evaluating what has gone before and envisaging what might be in order to respond appropriately. An attraction of moving to a reflective model was its dynamic developmental process which appeared to fit with the project's reflective approach.

The change process

Action research is characterised by a cyclical pattern of planning, acting, observing and reflecting (Webb 1989, Titchen & Binnie 1993). Elliot's spiral (Elliot 1981) was utilised as a relatively straightforward representation reflecting the idea of a continuing cycle of action-reflection steps. The action steps emerging through this study are summarised in Fig. 9.2.

To assist in the change process and to enable professional debate around the issues, four workshops were held in preparation for the change:

- An exploration of the nursing process
- Patient participation and patient empowerment
- Interpersonal skills development
- The process of action research

The workshops complimented an information pack and workbook where nurses were given the opportunity to critically review the proposal and to reflect on issues within it. Team meetings were held at regular intervals both before, during and after the implementation phase. Some staff were initially reluctant to offer any criticism or to speak about any problems they had encountered in this forum. This was

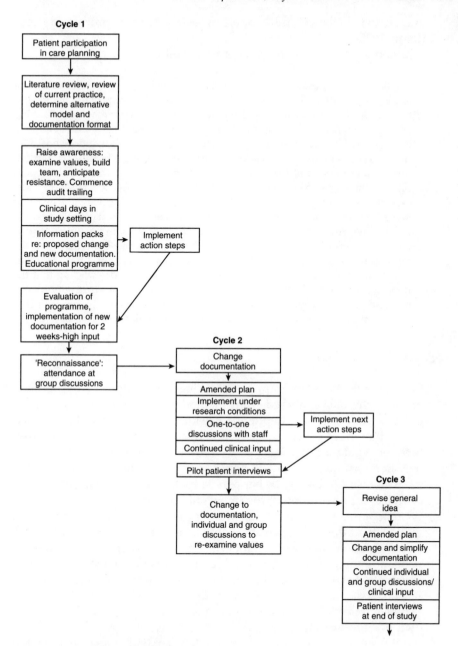

Fig. 9.2 Application of Elliot's spiral.

not a complete surprise; practitioners in this area, like many others, might be considered to have been socialised into an acceptance and compliance demanded by 'the organisation'. It would be crucial to the success of the project that they developed ownership, and this would only happen if nurses began to feel empowered. Structured reflection offered the challenge and support necessary for this process to occur (Johns 1995).

Julia offers some insight into her early feelings:

> The research proposal was greeted with mixed feelings by myself and the rest of the ward staff – excitement at being the ward chosen; fear of change and fear because of the focus of the research. Attitudes towards care planning among the staff varied; some saw the nursing process as 'just another chore' to be completed hurriedly at the end of a shift. 'Nobody reads it, it does not often relate to the patient', 'patients do not care about having a beautifully written care plan at the end of the bed if there is nobody to take them to the toilet'. Most of the negative comments regarding care planning came from the most experienced staff on the ward. This may stem from the way the nursing process was introduced and taught. The use of computerised care plans came in for some criticism from all grades of staff as time consuming, with only one terminal so staff had to queue to use it. However, despite the criticism of the nursing process, when the research asked us to stop using it, I felt like I was having the rug pulled out from under my feet and was discovering that the floor was no longer there. Whatever my feelings about the nursing process, I just could not see beyond it. Some of these feelings became apparent during the educational workshops prior to the implementation of the research.

Recognition of change

Changes which became apparent during the study will be outlined utilising the data gathered from methodological triangulation. Triangulation gave a greater depth and breadth to the study and addressed the limitations of previous research in this area. Allowing a comparison between what the nurses said they were doing (reflective journals), what they demonstrated they were doing (documentation review) and what the patients perceived to be happening (patient interviews) gave a more complete representation of the impact of change.

Content analysis of interview transcripts and reflective journals was guided by Burnard's thematic content analysis (Burnard 1991). The documentation analysis was undertaken by an expert panel who independently viewed and categorised identified patient concerns and who then looked at the way in which those concerns were reflected within the outcomes documented for each patient.

Julia's reflections offer a personal insight into the way in which her own practice was challenged during the study. She gives an account of the change process representing not only a personal transformation, but also a growing awareness and empowerment which enabled her (and others) to challenge organisational issues which impinged on practice.

The change

The areas of transformation are summarised as:

- Change from the view of patients' needs centred around 'activities of living' to a more holistic view and a move away from problem solving to mutual goal setting as the focus for planning care
- Recognition and challenging of 'emotional detachment'
- Recognition of the therapeutic nature of the nurse/patient relationship
- Enhancement of the named nurse concept

Change from the view of patients' needs centred around 'activities of living' to a more holistic view and a move away from problem solving to mutual goal setting as the focus for planning care

Julia noted: Care plans are less medically orientated and more holistic in nature with a greater emphasis on the concerns of the patient and their families.

The documentation review looked at the concerns elicited from patients with the aid of the Burford NDU Model's assessment framework (Johns 1994). It went on to determine how successfully those concerns had been translated into outcome statements, mutually arrived at with the patient. The analysis concluded that concerns were representative of patient concerns in 85% of cases. This fact, together with comments elicited from reflective journals, is supportive of the assessment framework in enabling patients to express their concerns and in offering a workable tool to nurses.

Considering the cue question, 'Who is this person?'

> Although I felt I had learned a great deal about Monty in the time that we had been chatting, I felt that I did not really 'know' him. This highlighted two points: firstly that the assessment would need to be ongoing right up until the point of discharge; secondly, do we ever 'know' someone and what does 'knowing someone' actually mean. This is not a criticism of the model but an observation on how this cue question could, was and is interpreted by some staff. We, as nurses, are socialised into thinking we 'know' someone only by their roles in society. For me, 'knowing' someone is much more than that. It is difficult to express just what it is. How this can be taught or learned is a difficult question. However, the ice was broken and we had many more conversations where we discussed our own beliefs and values and I felt that I got to know him better than I would previously have done.

The assessment framework was the one part of the research which was, from the outset, greeted with overwhelming enthusiasm. It is suggested that the cue questions offered by the framework became the precursor to change within individuals. Julia's reflections illustrate the way in which her practice was challenged through the demands of the framework, and the way in which guided reflection helped her through some difficult realisations:

The use of clinical supervision and reflection were crucial to the process of the transformation in practice, and remain so. It's difficult to envisage using the holistic model of assessment without guided reflection.

Julia's comments support the view of Johns & Graham (1996) that a 'coming together' of real life experience and espoused or desirable practice requires the space and structure offered within guided reflection.

Translating concerns into mutually negotiated goals with patients proved more difficult. In only half (54%) of the documentation analysed, the concerns identified by the patient were represented in the outcomes set. Where nurses were unable to elicit the patients' understanding of what was being asked, they appeared to resort to familiar care planning practices. The task of eliciting concerns and using strategies to enable the patient to translate and understand them as goals towards their recovery cannot be underestimated, highlighting the need for ongoing education and structured reflection in developing their interpersonal skills.

Recognition and challenging of 'emotional detachment'

Perhaps unsurprisingly, nurses were more easily able to identify outcomes and plan care around the more perceptible issues such as pain and sleep disturbance. Where concerns were related to the less tangible issues (i.e. fear, anxiety, low mood), nurses were less likely to represent these in outcome statements. 'Emotional detachment' is well-documented (Katz 1986; Holden 1990) and was recognised by one nurse within her journal:

> It's far more difficult ... you have to really get to know a person and give something of yourself which is hard when nurses often try to remain detached for their own sake.

Guided reflection is imperative as these defences begin to come to conscious awareness. Johns' (1995) model of structured reflection (see Fig. 1.1) provided the framework for Julia's supervision and the following reflections illustrate the way in which the processes of supervision, reflection and action research complemented each other:

> A gentleman was admitted to the ward. His bed was not ready, so whilst I was making his bed we chatted and continued to do so even when the bed was finished, which was an achievement for me. Through previous clinical supervision sessions it became evident that I always needed a physical prop to enable me to begin to interact with patients. This was a shield to protect the inner me from the potential hurt of 'getting involved'. Before clinical supervision, I had found myself almost at burnout point. I had a fear of becoming involved with my patients; I would wear my uniform as though it were a suit of armour. On stepping into this armour, I became 'robo-nurse' and the real me was cocooned inside. I had this perception because prior to clinical

supervision, no support mechanisms were available and to some extent 'getting involved' was not encouraged.

Exploration stimulated by the cue question: 'How does this patient make me feel', became a crucial point in Julia's journey:

I felt comfortable with Monty at first. Then he started to ask me questions about myself and my home life. I could feel the panic starting to rise. This is where the part of my mind which seemed to be hovering above me and analysing the situation came to the fore. What was the panic about? I felt that he was breaking through my invisible barriers! I almost cut the conversation dead and felt this overwhelming urge to get out the previous model of assessment, to take charge and to start filling in the little boxes with inane statements.

My fears started to surface during my initial clinical supervision meetings. As I started to examine my interactions with my patients, it became clear that I consciously avoided forming any sort of relationship with the majority of them. When I did interact with my patients, it was during, and often initiated by a particular nursing action, such as giving an injection, and it often ended when the action was complete. After completion of the interpersonal skills workshop, it became clear that I would need to examine and reflect upon my previous interactions. I was certain that I had the skills being discussed, there just seemed to be a barrier which was preventing me from using them and developing caring, meaningful and fulfilling relationships with my patients.

Guided reflection through clinical supervision enabled Julia to bring her defences to conscious awareness and to begin to challenge them:

I started to 'know myself' through the following situation:
Jack had a chronic illness, he had been cared for on the ward on several occasions and for long periods. I was his primary nurse and we had a close relationship. It was a very busy period on the ward. I had learned that Jack had been admitted to one of the other wards. I instigated his return to my ward so that he could continue his care with the medical and nursing staff that knew him and that he was familiar with. It was at this time that a colleague raised the point that this would probably be Jack's last admission. She questioned how I and the other nurses in the team would deal with this? I must be honest, I chose to ignore the question. On his return to the ward, I found that Jack was different. He required a lot of physical care that he had not required before. He became very demanding, always using the call buzzer or shouting for assistance; even though we were spending a great deal of time with him, he would call us seconds after we had left the room. Jack's constant demands for attention were putting a strain on our relationship, added to which it became implied that the nursing care he was receiving was lacking. I felt that I was giving him everything I could give of myself. I became very upset and angry ... very angry. I felt that I had been stabbed in the back by an old friend. Our relationship quickly deteriorated to the point that I told him what I felt about his behaviour.

The situation was brought to clinical supervision and following a long and tearful session with my supervisor, I was able to verbalise to her what was deep down, that I couldn't face up to the fact that he was dying. It was a painful process and I felt ashamed, particularly of the confrontation I had had with Jack. Following the session, I needed to act. I went into Jack and told him that I still cared for him and I apologised for the things I had said. I also told him that I was scared about losing him. We both cried and hugged. Later that evening a member of staff called me at home to tell me that Jack had died peacefully in his wife's arms that evening.

Why had this situation arisen? There was a part of me that always had to be right. I did not heed the warning given to me by my colleague when I was arranging for Jack to return to the ward. This is one of the most unsatisfactory aspects of my self that I have discovered. I can see this 'know it all' trait in myself now. I had a lack of knowledge about the psychological effects of dying and I was unable to recognise early enough this lack of knowledge. I wanted Jack to be the same person as I had known before, for the relationship to be as easy as it was before. I acted in the way that I did towards Jack following the suggestion that his care was lacking, in order to exert my power over him. I took the criticisms very personally without analysing why they might have occurred. I acted defensively. I was reluctant to face up to the fact that Jack was dying – my fear of losing someone who had become dear to me.

Julia concludes:

Using reflection has helped me to find out more about myself. Reflection has been and at times remains a painful process of discovery. However, it has its rewards. Today I no longer feel like robo-nurse. I have the confidence to let the real me shine out.

Recognition of the therapeutic nature of the nurse/patient relationship

Julia noted: 'Some nurses have stated that they feel closer to their patients'.

One of the categories derived from the analysis of the reflective journals was that of 'rapport'. Within all of the journals, reflections identified changes in the way nurses were interacting with patients, feelings of greater satisfaction with the relationship and a greater sense of informality within the relationship. Rapport was linked with participation and involvement. Where rapport did not exist within the relationship, it appeared that patients were less likely to feel involved. Patients appeared to value what *they* defined as the informality of the approach of nurses, demonstrated within one of the categories arising from the analysis of patient interviews: 'friendliness of approach'. Here, patients spoke about feeling comfortable, at ease and able to ask questions which were readily answered. Indeed, while more questions were raised than answered in terms of what patients understood by 'involvement' and participation, it was apparent that involvement was viewed by patients as being linked with the ability to ask questions. The feeling of involvement seemed to generate from the approach of nurses who gave permission for them to ask questions, either directly or indirectly, through their friendliness and informality. This at least appears to offer the groundwork for the development of therapeutic relationships and support for a holistic model where the nature of care is predominantly concerned with the relationship between the nurse and the patient (Johns 1994).

> We talked about him and I started to go through the cue questions in my mind, not directly asking him, but trying to use them in the conversation we were having. The effect was amazing. It was as though I was really thinking for the first time about what I was doing and why; my mind went into overdrive – this was exciting. Whilst keeping the cue questions at the front of my mind, I was keeping the conversation flowing and analysing the whole situation at the same time. And he asked me questions about me! Highlighting the fact that he perceived the interaction as a conversation rather than an interview.

Enhancement of the named nurse concept

> The named nurse concept has been more rigorously implemented. Both the patients and their relatives are more aware of who their named nurse is and what this means. Introductions of the nurses coming on to the shift are made to patients and there is a formal 'handing over' of patients from one nurse to another when staff are going to be away for long periods of time.

Some of the limitations

The transformations in nurses and the way that nurses were practising can be seen as subtle changes in their 'way of being'. I, perhaps like many, started out with the mistaken belief that I could change the world. To tackle the issues of care planning and patient participation over such a limited period can be seen as ambitious at the very least.

There were many dangers in the approach, which were only partly understood and confronted at the beginning of the process. Perhaps the most controversial for advocates of action research was the way in which the area of concern was chosen. It could be argued that any change introduced in this way by a relative 'outsider' would be short-lived and ownership by the participants problematic. Ensuring ownership was therefore crucial to the success of the project. It is tentatively suggested that ownership was achieved; the work continues a year later without my direct input and this is a tribute to the work of the nurses on the ward and their commitment.

The second danger, borne out in the early stages of the research, was that the change would be viewed simply as a documentation change over and above a cultural, attitudinal and philosophical development. Six weeks into the implementation phase of the study, the researcher's personal journal reflects:

> 'I am despondent at the quality of what is being written. It seems that the way of writing has not yet changed, signifying a lack of any

conceptual shift. The nurses seem to be repeating old care-planning practices onto new documentation. Desired outcomes are written as nurse identified problems, they are neither measurable nor patient focused, rather they continue to reflect the medical model...'

Personal supervision and further reflection were crucial to me in translating despondence into a stepping stone for the next action steps. Of course, this was a vital moment. It was anticipated at the outset that the approach of the nurses would change so dramatically that the patients would experience something different on this ward. It was hoped that some insight would be gained into the desire of patients for participation because they would experience the invitation to partici-pate. It is considered a failing of previous work in this area, where patients were asked about participation without ever having been given the chance to experience it (Waterworth & Luker 1990).

However, two months into the study, it was apparent that the aim was again somewhat ambitious in the light of the way in which nurses continued to document care. It was to take far longer than the three months allowed for the implementation for the cultural changes to be significant enough to impact greatly on care delivery. Having said this, during the final stages of the study, there was evidence that some patients were experiencing the invitation to participate. A further cate-gory derived from the journal transcripts was labelled 'improving'. Nurses themselves were able to reflect on how arduous they had found the change. As they became more familiar with the documentation, they were able to focus on developing skills which would facilitate greater involvement of patients. I noted in my journal my realisation that a philosophical shift had taken place, when one nurse, during super-vision, commented that she felt that the art of nursing had been put back into her practice, relating it to a greater depth within the relationships she was able to form with patients.

Conclusion

It is concluded that the therapeutic nature of the nurse/patient rela-tionship was demonstrated within this study. Utilising the Burford NDU Model: Caring in Practice (Johns 1994) proved to be an effective structure to enable nurses to 'know' the patient more holistically and in turn elicit *their* concerns on coming into the ward.

The processes of action research, clinical supervision and reflective practice complemented each other in bringing together theory and research in an attempt to challenge previous practice of arguable merit. Through facilitation, nurses became empowered and able to value their interactions as a therapeutic resource. A very real difference to their practice was demonstrated with the nurses themselves controlling the change and deciding the way forward. This contrasts vividly with a culture where more and more practice is dictated by processes imposed on nurses from outside.

The use of reflective practice as a tool of research is relatively new. This study has demonstrated that reflective practice is not only a valuable and valid method of data collection, but also a means by which nurses develop through a critical examination of their practice. Through the giving of self and the development of rapport within the nurse patient relationship, that relationship can be seen to have been strengthened, making it meaningful and satisfying to both nurses and patients.

References

Benner, P. & Tanner, C. (1987) How expert nurses use initiation. *American Journal of Nursing,* 12, 23–31.

Boyd, E.M. & Fales, A.W. (1983) Reflecting learning: key to learning from experience. *Journal of Humanistic Psychology,* **23**(2), 99–117.

Burnard, P. (1991) A method of analysing interview transcripts in qualitative research. *Nurse Education Today,* **11**, 461-46.

Butterworth, T., Carson, J., White, E., Jeacock, J. & Clements, A. (1996) *It's good to talk?* The twenty-three site evaluation project of clinical supervision in England and Scotland: an interim report. University of Manchester.

Carr, W. & Kemmis, S. (1986) *Becoming Critical: Education, Knowledge and Action Research.* The Falmer Press, London.

CURN Project (1982) *Mutual goal setting in patient care.* Conduct & Utilisation of Research in Nursing Project, Michigan Nurses Association. Grune & Stratton, London.

Davis, B.D., Billings, J.R. & Ryland, R.K. (1994) Evaluation of nursing process documentation. *Journal of Advanced Nursing,* **19**, 960–68.

Elliot, J. (1981) see McNiff, J. 1992, pp. 29-30.

Fonteyn, M.E. & Cooper, L.F. (1994) The written nursing process: is it still useful to nursing education? *Journal of Advanced Nursing,* **19**, 315–19.

Ford, P. & Walsh, M. (1994) *New Rituals for Old: Nursing through the Looking Glass.* Butterworth Heinemann, London.

Henderson, V. (1982) The nursing process – is the title right? *Journal of Advanced Nursing,* **7**, 103–109.

Holden, R. (1990) Models, muddles and medicine. *International Journal of Nursing Studies,* **27**(3), 223–34.

Holter, I.M. & Schwartz-Barcott, D. (1993) Action research: what is it? How has it been used and how can it be used in nursing? *Journal of Advanced Nursing,* **18**, 298–304.

Johns, C. (1994) *The Burford NDU Model: Caring in Practice.* Blackwell Science, Oxford.

Johns, C. (1995) Framing learning through reflection within Carper's fundamental ways of knowing in nursing. *Journal of Advanced Nursing,* **22**, 226–34.

Johns, C. & Graham, J. (1996) Using a reflective model of nursing and guided reflection. *Nursing Standard,* **11**(2), 34–8.

Katz, J. (1986) *The Silent World of Doctor and Patient.* Free Press, New York.

Koch, T. (1994) Beyond measurement: fourth generation evaluation in nursing. *Journal of Advanced Nursing,* **20**, 1148–55.

Luker, K.A. (1992) Research and development in nursing (guest editorial). *Journal of Advanced Nursing,* **17**, 1151–2.

Mathews, M. (1980) The Marxist theory of schooling: a study of epistemology and education. In *Becoming Critical: Education, Knowledge and Action Research* (1986) (W. Carr & S. Kemmis), pp. 181. The Falmer Press, London.

McHugh, M. (1986) Nursing process: musings on the methods. *Holistic Nursing Practice,* **1**(1), 21–8.

McNiff, J. (1988) *Action Research: Principles and Practice.* Macmillan, London.

Palmer, P.N. (1988) Nursing care plans: are we protecting sacred cows or beating dead horses? (editorial). *Association of Operating Room Nurses Journal,* **47**(6), 1357–8.

Shea, H.L. (1986) A conceptual framework to study the use of nursing care plans. *International Journal of Nursing Studies,* **23**(2), 147–57.

Sovie, M.D. (1988) Clinical nursing practices and patient outcomes: evaluation, evolution, and revolution. (Legitimizing radical change to maximize nurses' time for quality care). *Nursing Economics,* **7**(2), 79–85.

Taylor-Gwozdz, D. & Del-Tongo Armanasco, V. (1992) Streamlining patient care documentation. *Journal of Nursing Administration,* **22**(5), 35–9.

Titchen, A. & Binnie, A. (1993) Research partnerships: collaborative action research in nursing. *Journal of Advanced Nursing,* **18**, 858–65.

Trnobranski, P.H. (1994) Nurse-patient negotiation: assumption or reality? *Journal of Advanced Nursing,* 1994, **19**, 733–7.

Waterworth, S. & Luker, K.A. (1990) Reluctant collaborators: do patients want to be involved in decisions concerning care? *Journal of Advanced Nursing,* **15**, 971–6.

Webb, C. (1989) Action research: philosophy, methods and personal experiences. *Journal of Advanced Nursing,* **14**, 403–10.

Chapter 10

Understanding the Nature of Nursing Through Reflection: a Case Study Approach

Iain Graham

Introduction

This chapter describes the process of two reflective cycles, based upon the method of new paradigm research, which two groups of nurses followed in an attempt to clarify the nature of their nursing practice. The need for knowledge which is specific to the practice of nursing has been recognised since the beginning of modern nursing. Florence Nightingale wrote, 'I believe ... that the very elements of nursing are all but unknown ... are as little understood for the well as for the sick. The same laws of health or of nursing, for they are in reality the same, obtain among the well as among the sick' (Nightingale 1859, p. 6).

She went on to argue that nursing knowledge has become increasingly confused with the knowledge of pathology. In an attempt to try and clear such confusion, she clarified what she believed to be the knowledge base of medicine and the knowledge base of nursing. This resulted in the statement that the aim and purpose of nursing, 'was to put the patient in the best condition for nature to act upon him' (Nightingale 1859, p. 74). In reading the work of Nightingale, one can accept her argument as to the purpose of nursing practice, and assume the charge that she gave nurses.

This chapter is to present how some nurses enquired into how they did put the patient that they cared for in the best condition for nature to cure them. My role was to facilitate this enquiry and to provide academic leadership in the form of helping them to interpret the nature of their practice by co-ordinating an enquiry process.

If our practice is to become based on sound knowledge discovered through research, then it is essential that we enter, in Schön's (1987) words, 'the swampy lowland, messy confusing problems defy technical solution' (p. 3) in order to map it out and interpret its meanings. The nurses in this reflective enquiry decided that they needed to undertake this type of work. They knew that the positivist science paradigm was inadequate for their purpose and therefore approached me for help in their endeavours within a different type of research paradigm.

The model of research I offered them was based upon the work of Reason and Rowan (1981) and Reason (1988), and is termed new paradigm research. The central tenet of the new paradigm is collaboration between researcher and researched when conducting the enquiry. All involved in the enquiry collaborate in the quest for knowledge, becoming in fact co-enquirers. The work therefore becomes not only a research form but also a method of education, personal development and social action. In essence the co-enquirers work together to:

(1) Discuss the research area
(2) Decide on the methods of the enquiry
(3) Observe themselves as the enquirers and the subjects
(4) Reflect upon their experience of learning and developing
(5) Decide together on the resolution of any problems encountered
(6) Decide the action to be taken once the findings have come to light.

This collaborative enquiry method became attractive to the nurses involved as it provided them with a means of investigating the nature of 'the swampy lowlands' by illuminating their practice through the medium of reflection. This would enable each of the nurses to observe themselves, reflect upon experiences gained, learn from that reflection and acknowledge their personal development needs.

Background

The nurses involved in the reflective cycles came from two distinct groups. One group consisted of twelve medical nurses who worked in an acute general medical ward. The other consisted of ten psychiatric nurses who worked in an assessment ward for the elderly mentally ill. The two groups did not come together for the enquiry; they were quite distinctive, following their respective lines of enquiry quite independently. Both groups had been acknowledged by the Kings Fund as nursing development units (NDU). Freeman (1996), for the Kings Fund, defines a nursing development unit as a 'clinical area which has a challenging and questioning culture. The NDU should strive to achieve improvements in order to develop nursing practice and evaluate new approaches to patient care.' Indeed, both groups of nurses aspired to the hope that such an activity would bring their philosophy of care to life and help them develop their nursing practice so as to improve the quality of care to their patients.

Reflective practice

I steered my clinical colleagues to consider their lived experiences of nursing as encapsulated by the notion of phenomenological reflection. The purpose of phenomenological reflection is to try and grasp the essential meaning of something. Van Manen (1990, p. 77) argues that this is both an easy and difficult task to do, because there is a difference between our pre-reflective lived-in understanding and our reflective grasp of the phenomenological structure of the lived experience: 'To get at the latter is a difficult and often laborious task'. The insight into the essence of what a phenomenon such as nursing is, involves a process of reflectively seizing a situation, of clarifying it and of making explicit the structural meaning of the lived experience in terms of themes or constructs. Ultimately the goal of phenomenological reflection and explication is to effect a more direct contact with the experience as lived. In other words, the challenging questions within nursing practice found within the swampy lowlands are often difficult to define and are often of an emotive nature – issues of the human experience and condition concerning the intimate nature of birth and death, of coping and of dying, of living with chronic illness and emotional despair or mental deterioration.

The description developed from the two groups of nurses' reflection would be grounded therefore within the experience that the nurse and patient were currently having, and it is from this that the substance of nursing can be named. I believe that what we were trying to do was to put the patient in the best condition for nature to cure them, by interpreting and examining the human condition as experienced and known by both the nurse and the patient through the process of the nursing practice. A common theme that emerged through my preliminary discussions with both nursing groups was that the nurses stated that they often intuitively did things in order to provide the patients with some sort of care before they fully understood what they were doing. The goal therefore of the reflective work was to try and identify this unknown area of practice.

The beginning

I met with both the teams for an afternoon workshop to explore the nature of reflective practice and to develop ground rules by which we could run a co-operative enquiry group. I also spent time in each of the clinical areas before the workshop in order to experience the culture. My personal experience of facilitating group learning has taught me that during the initial stages, being able to raise concrete examples of practice helps group members to focus attention and articulate their viewpoint. The purpose behind this was to ground reflective activity in a purposeful and actively directed way and not simply allow idle meanderings or day-dreaming to occur. The ground rules were common to any group work activity, featuring issues of group responsibility, confidentiality and mutual respect.

I felt it important that the two groups should have some consensus as regards the goals, norms, roles and other aspects of the group functioning in order to feel more at ease. The reasons for this were that the medical nurses had no experience of group work and therefore felt somewhat daunted by the prospect of entering into such a close and intimate process of learning and developing. The psychiatric nurses, on the other hand, had experience of group work, but I was keen to establish that this type of group would be fundamentally different from the psycho-therapeutic groups that they facilitated in their everyday work. I was aware that the existence of dynamic forces within group work, be they intra-personal, inter-personal or environmental, do operate to either facilitate or inhibit the groups' performance.

Emden (1991, cited in Gray and Pratt) draws attention to the personal processes involved when engaging in reflective work. She says that one becomes acutely aware of one's actions, thoughts and feelings within a complex milieu of people and events, and that when you comment on the other's behaviour you may indeed illuminate as much about your-self as of them. This was the fundamental aspect of the workshop activity. Gaining an acknowledgement from each group member of their personal responsibility to achieve the task of identifying and interpret-ing their practice, was dependent upon them each making an individual journey, by reflection, into their practice and then sharing that indivi-dual journey with their colleagues.

We discussed at length how they would deal with their feelings of vulnerability and embarrassment, anger and guilt as well as their feel-ings of joy and elation as they described their individual journeys through the reflective enquiry. We also discussed how we, as colleagues and co-enquirers, would be supportive to each other when these feelings occurred and what we could do to enable the feelings to be dealt with satisfactorily. Members knew that they would be revealing their indi-vidual practice strategies to colleagues for the first time and this can often be a potentially frightening situation. Nurses have been socialised to be emotionally withdrawn from patients, and it only with the advent of new nursing (Salvage 1984) that the nurse/patient relationship and the behaviour and communication that exists and grows between nurse and patient has become acknowledged. I believe that nurses are terrified of being made to look foolish or inadequate and that the concept of the cool and competent clinical nurse is a stereotype that is reluctant to die. The stereotype will not die if nurses hesitate in exploring the swampy lowlands of their practice.

The cycle of reflection

The period of reflection lasted for over a year for both groups and consisted of three phases of activity. Each phase consisted of a three month period with the group assembling for 90 minutes every two weeks, after which an evaluation activity took place. The evaluation consisted of interviewing the members of the group with the aim of trying to get an appreciation of how the process of reflection was aiding their practice in terms of clarification and description. The three phases were:

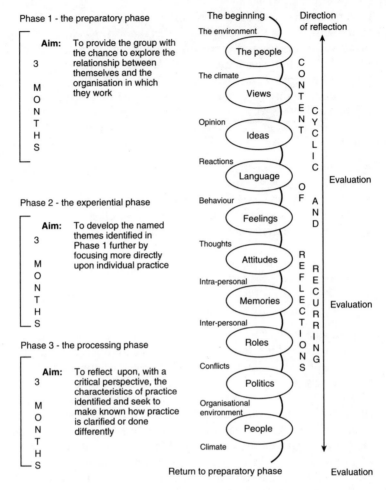

Fig. 10.1 The cycle of reflection.

(1) A preparatory phase in which the individual considers the demands of the experiences ahead and the resources required
(2) An experiential phase in which practice occurs
(3) A processing phase in which the preceding events are reconstructed in order to make sense of them

Phase 1 – the preparatory phase

The aim of this phase was to provide the group with the opportunity to explore the relationship between themselves and the organisation in which they work. Phase 1 was rather prescriptive because my concern about group work dynamics and the need to ground the demands and experiences ahead in a holding structure. I had the support of my co-enquirers that phase 1 should be purposeful and actively directed toward a goal, and therefore in keeping with Van Manen's (1994) statement, 'as we examine situations taken from real life ... the way to bring examples to reflective understanding is to fix them'. I endeavoured to facilitate each group by reflective debate which sought to help the two groups of nurses to fix for themselves their relationship with their social reality of nursing. Buckenham and McGrath's (1983) investigation into the social reality of nurses provided me with ten characteristics to focus the nurses' reflection on their real life experiences. The characteristics were:

- Historical perspectives
- Nature of our nursing
- The education system to prepare us for our role
- The theoretical underpinnings to our practice
- Professional and personal accountability
- Ethical concerns
- Professional culture
- Professional ideology
- Quality of practice
- Purpose of caring

In practice, often one topic would be related to another and would spill over from one group into the next, thereby giving a dynamic interplay of concepts and ideas. These debates became very lively and stimulating as my colleagues settled into the routine of discussing their social reality. The debate, which often had the similarities of an encounter group (Rogers 1970), revealed numerous themes which underpinned the social reality of both teams' nursing practice. In both settings, responsibility, job purpose, autonomy, power and focus of activity became the central concepts around which a picture of the nature of their nursing emerged. Perhaps the most important concept to emerge from phase 1 was the realisation that they, as nurses, were somehow fundamentally engaged in the activity of nursing. This may seem strange to the reader at first sight, but it is suggesting that the nurses in both groups slowly began to realise that they had some accountability and responsibility in the provision of the type of nursing they wished to practice, in their respective areas. This is perhaps best encapsulated by one nurse who works on the medical ward, who said, 'when they realised that this lady was going to die, I realised my responsibility for the first time with regard to the type of nursing I wished to have practised on that ward. I realised that I was the one who needed to hold the woman's hand as she died, that this was not going to be given to anybody else, and that her comfort, her need was in my hands, and my hands alone'.

The realisation by the nurses that they had a crucial role to play in patient care and were not simply there to carry out hospital functioning or service the medical profession was beginning to be made. With this realisation came a further insight: that their nursing was rather invisible. No-one knew what nursing actually was; the patients, the clients, relatives and other health professionals all had a view as to what nursing was about, but the real nursing, like the holding of the hand of someone dying, was invisible, and was not given high status within the total healthcare system. This concept of invisibility was something that Lawler (1991, p. 224) describes in detail in her work. She says that patients often do not talk about the nurses or the nursing care they receive, because it is intimately involved in the way their body works and how they presented themselves as individuals at a time of vulnerability and need. The concept of invisibility was a recurring theme.

The nurses in both NDU's were aiming to provide individualised care. Yet what they were realising was that the preparation they had received in their training had been totally inadequate in preparing them to provide individualised care. So not only was it invisible, but they were totally ill-prepared to do what they did in an emotionally satisfying way for both the patient and themselves. This I thought was intriguing, remembering that one goal of the reflective cycle was to try to understand what the nurses did before they did it. One can remember being told in nursing school to reassure the patient, often over and over again. To reassure them of what and how? This was never explained. In an attempt to provide individualised care, the nurses did reassure, but it was only through the medium of the group that their methods of reassuring came to light, and for the first time they were explaining to each other how they engaged in this type of nursing practice.

As soon as the discussion within each of the reflective groups began to raise such issues for debate, other insights into how each of the nurses did their work began to be made. For example, they had always expected and assumed that they were very supportive towards each other, and were able to empathise regularly with their colleagues. Through the medium of the reflective activity they were becoming aware that perhaps they were not as supportive as they professed to be, nor as honest with each other as perhaps they should be. They were beginning to realise that they worked in a climate of fantasy at times, where they had made assumptions and speculations on how each of them worked, and now they were being confronted with the fact that what they believed to be good or competent practice in colleagues was perhaps not as good or as competent as first assumed.

All of these dynamics needed to be facilitated and steered by myself, so that a feeling of positiveness and benevolence could emerge. The facilitation required careful managing because individual group members began to confront other members in a direct and potentially embarrassing way, emotions sometimes ran high and tempers flared.

Phase 2 – the experiential phase

The aim here was to further develop the named themes identified in phase 1 by focusing more directly upon individual practice. Therefore the process moved to individual group members reflecting on patient care which they shared within the group, and leading a discussion on what they had learnt about the care they had given. The nurse would also present aspects of literature to stimulate debate and discussion. So, for example, if they were talking about a patient with HIV and Aids they might well interject current theoretical commentary from the literature and compare and contrast the literature to the care that they were giving or had given to the patient in their care.

The debate within the presentation was less philosophical and ideo-logical than in phase 1. It was also less confrontational and it was noted that the content of the reflections had recurring themes and concepts, such as the behaviour of certain patients or the memories nurses held from their experience. Group members provided feedback and would often also give praise and support as they heard their colleague reveal aspects of their work, attitudes, beliefs and views about nursing, per-haps for the first time in that type of setting. Members were encouraged to make suggestions with regard to the care they had heard being pre-sented; they might well provide their own experiences of caring for such a person, thereby fostering personal development of their colleagues as well as themselves in how to problem solve, manage risk taking or with regard to giving competent, appropriate nursing care.

From these presentations a number of areas of practice were identified that were significant to each of the unit's overall nursing activity. The nurse/patient relationship was something that was reviewed constantly when presented within each of the care studies. Within this aspect such issues as closeness and intimacy between nurse and patient were topics of debate. One nurse, for example, talked about how deeply moved they were by the sudden death of a patient they were caring for, while another talked about how she felt jealous of the relationship the patient had with her life partner. The feeling that somehow she, the nurse, was being displaced by the patient's husband, when trying to provide care for someone with Alzheimer's, led to an interesting debate about the position of the nurse within a family unit.

The concept of primacy was another area of dialogue. Who holds primacy in nursing? They often debated at length, as they presented each of the care studies, just what their level of accountability was. Was it the consultant, the hospital system, the clinical directorate or they themselves held primacy for nursing care? They knew the rhetoric, they knew that in theory they were accountable for what they did, but they also knew that they would only obtain vicarious liability by the hospital if they practised their nursing within the hospital rules, pro-cedures and policies. If they chose not to do so, that opened them up to risk, and this was a constant area of discussion as we discussed each case each week. Some nurses talked at length about how their growing confidence and ability were moving them away from the policies and procedures of the hospital and into truly negotiated patient care. This was often in the case when patients were 'given up', as described by one group member, by the doctors of the hospital, and the patient became acknowledged as a 'nursing only case'. The nurses at this point would have to deal with the concept of failure – failure to cure, to heal, to return the patient to his life – and this required them to alter perspectives of the care given so that it was not seen as a failure on anyone's part. This was a major area of discussion.

Their feelings and personal beliefs about nursing were revealed within this second phase of reflection. Some members were content to present a more stereotypical view that the nurse was really a doctor's assistant and carried out only the orders and prescriptions of care as deemed appropriate to their status. Others felt that nursing had more potential, and that nurses could work in a much more expanded way than within the confines of the hospital policy. This created some distance between certain members of the groups and it was something that had to be managed by good facilitation, and yet it also focused members on their inter-personal relationships within the team.

Another key concept that emerged from phase 2 was that of advocacy, in particular on the medical ward. This team of nurses talked about inappropriate admissions: that the ward was quite 'a high tech unit' with lots of machinery involved in patient care, and yet occasionally they would have patients admitted to them who required a different type of intensive care nursing. For example, some patients might be confused or had suffered permanent brain damage due to a viral infection. These patients would wander about the ward, would interfere with other patients and their care, and would be conceived as irritating by the nursing team. At first the nurses would become irritated themselves, but when one of the nurses presented one such patient, they began to formulate a better picture of their advocacy responsibilities. They realised that this patient was not really being cared for, that they were being 'warehoused' and that they should be better placed in a different type of environment, and that they as nurses had something to say and do about that.

Such examples of care began to make the team question what intensive care nursing is. Is intensive care nursing involved in the observation of and interaction with somebody who is confused, or is intensive care nursing involved with people who are wired up to machines? Is intensive care nursing defined by nurses or by medicine? The presentations raised more questions than answers, but what was also emerging was a skill set to the knowledge base that these nurses in both NDUs needed in order to enable their nature of nursing to come to life and for them to feel competent and positive about their role as nurses.

It was at the second stage evaluation that both groups were able to articulate their respective conceptual frameworks of practice; to clarify what they had to do to put the person in the best condition for nature to cure; and to say what activities, behaviours or values had to be displayed. They were establishing their own bedrock which gave them strength and conviction as to what their nursing was all about.

The medical ward's conceptual framework of practice

To the nurses on the medical ward the over-riding philosophical concept that underpinned their view of their role and activity and purpose was concerned with their understanding of sickness. The patients that they worked with were sick; they had major disease and illness which was life threatening and required sophisticated medical intervention and nursing care in order to enable the patients to attain some level of health homeostasis. The reflective process enabled the nurses to move their understanding of sickness away from the medical diagnosis and pathology, and to see the patients as either suffering from stress and disease or pain and disease, which had altered the patients' perceptions of themselves and their life and their relationships. They might have been enduring illness which occurred in acute phases, or they might be in crisis, not just physiological crisis but emotional, intellectual, spiritual and social as well. This way of seeing their patient led to understanding what they needed to do as nurses. They knew they had to facilitate a sense of 'coping for their patients', that the patients themselves would need to feel comforted, feel supported, feel that they were benefiting from their stay in the hospital environment. The nurses also knew they would have to facilitate a sense of reprieve, that certain aspects of the lifestyle and behaviour of the patient would need to be 'put on hold', with the nurse somehow holding the balance. Therefore to provide balance was a major aspect of the nursing purpose on the medical ward.

To understand how the nurses would provide a sense of coping, reprieve and balance in the context of the sickness, one needs to appreciate how the nurses themselves understood the concept of 'self as a nurse' with regard to the needs of the patients they were working with. This required sophisticated understandings in terms of self-awareness, self-concept, role clarity, personal experience, belief and value system. The nurses expressed in each of their case studies that to maintain the sense of person as an individual required the nurses to know the patient vis-a-vis the nurse as a person. This infusion required the nurses to develop experiential knowledge based on their instincts and intuitions as a means of determining how the process of nursing was managed and delivered. They all admitted that sometimes this personal involvement, this insight based on their own self-concept, did not work; the patient presented in such a macabre or strange way that the nurse could find no relationship to their own particular lifestyle and that required greater involvement by the nurse.

Gradually through each of the reflective sessions we became aware that as each of the presentations took place the themes that were emerging as characteristics of nursing within the medical ward were being identified. These were:

(1)   Mopper-upper
(2)   Referrer identifier

(3) Specialist specific skill
(4) Coupling

Only 'mopper-upper ' and coupling will be described here. The nurses described how on a day to day basis they would 'mop-up' all sorts of aspects involved in the human condition of their patients. They would not just 'mop-up' the system, i.e. ensure that the patient gets their investigations done on time, that they see the doctor when needed, or ensure that social workers or family members are attended to. They also 'mopped-up' aspects of the human condition which were not so obvious or visible. For these things, such as helplessness, boredom, anger or inability, the nurse would act as some sort of sponge. They would also apply this 'mopping-up' activity to relatives and other health professionals, somehow making everything 'all right' so that the world could continue in its seemingly unchaotic way.

Coupling, which somehow embraces its sexual connotation as well, was the means by which the nurse became attached or perhaps not attached to the patients and their care – how some patients could never become attached to the nurse, because they frightened the nurse or the patient's condition frightened the nurse, because the nurse felt unskilled or inadequate to deal with it. But when the nurse felt able to deal with whatever was being presented, this unique self-reference model came into play and the coupling that took place was powerful, dynamic and courageous and the nurse could achieve a lot for the benefit of the patient. These characteristics were displayed in the way the nurses carried out their activity of practice by 'supporting', 'empowering', 'facilitating' and 'doing'.

The psychiatric ward's conceptual framework of practice
The starting point for nursing practice on the psychiatric ward stems from an understanding of client centred therapy and the world of therapeutics, i.e. consisting of a humanistic framework which undergrids the nursing process within the NDU. The emphasis of the care was on understanding the psycho-social processes as a basis for understanding emotional/psychiatric illness, although acknowledgement of biological processes was also there.

Their over-riding philosophy was based on understanding the feelings of people, and stopping the feelings of people from being minimised in an increasingly controlling medical environment. The nurses believed strongly that feelings, attitudes, values and beliefs, which embodied the presentation of the individual person, were very important to their understanding of their role as nurses in this particular setting. These were fundamental to keeping the sense of 'humanness' or personal identity apparent within the patient, and to acknowledging the social being and that social groups and processes were very important in maintaining that sense of 'humanness'. Therefore the purpose of nursing evolved around the nurses' ability to fully perceive the humanness of their patients as well as perceive their own sense of 'humanness'.

As with my description of development on the medical ward, the nurses identified significant characteristics of their relationships with patients, which were explored for their meaning and developed.

Phase 3 – the processing phase

The aim of phase 3 was to reflect upon and further explore from a critical perspective the defined characteristics of practice that we had uncovered, and to seek how we would do things differently. We sought to further clarify purpose and understanding of the lived experiences of nursing, and to articulate meaning to that lived experience. From my own position I was very aware that we had been engaging in a process of self-consciousness raising in which we had been looking critically at the traditions that had guided our activity. Thompson (1985) thinks it increasingly important that nurses do engage in such activity and engage in a process of rational deliberation, such as critical enquiry. Allen, who also wrote in 1985, suggests that critical theory generation in nursing offers nurses the opportunity to shatter the ideological mirror that traps them and their clients in any particular situation. Critical enquiry forces nurses to question the status quo at every turn. The sifting and sorting through via reflection of personal and working lives may enable nurses to formulate a truly alternative view of practice and themselves.

Generally, both teams had raised their awareness of what it meant to be nurses in these environments. In both areas, working as a team with improving communication systems was better understood. We had identified and described what had been hitherto disguised nursing practices. By being able to talk about being a 'mopper-upper' or a 'change-maker', we were able to utilise this emancipatory knowledge (Fay 1987) to better engage and plan patient care and to communicate that care to other members of the multi-disciplinary team. We now had what Heron (1992, p. 157, p. 180) would call 'practical knowledge' of the work of nursing, and were now all well able to articulate the nature of that work.

I believe that this is best testified by considering an evaluation by one of the group members. Peter was a patient who had received medical care for liver failure. As his condition stabilised the nurses focused their attention on more acutely ill people, and began to ignore Peter. Nesta, the nurse responsible for his care, acknowledged in her presentation that she had focused so much on the medical need of the patient that she had forgotten his nursing needs and therefore his needs as a fellow human being.

She commented:

What would I have done differently? Two aspects of nursing have always remained constant: the need to care and the need to communicate. Peter, my patient, was often lonely in a crowded ward. He suffered from the loss of casual chat, which can often cause a major and distressing deprivation. The failure to communicate causes more suffering than any other problem, except when relieving pain. We were all guilty of depriving Peter of good communication. We were all guilty of paternalism by interfering with Peter's liberty which affected his welfare, needs, happiness and interests. The need to talk to Peter and explain things was my firm responsibility and the failure to do so did him harm. I believe I was guilty of causing Peter harm in this way by sometimes bowing to pressure from his relatives and partner. If I were to do anything different it would have to be to remember I am accountable and responsible to my patient; I must always put them first.

In being involved in the situation, by being aware of the components of the situation and then by examining my responses, I believe I have become increasingly more effective in my work by the knowledge gained through reflective practice. It enables me to focus the needs of patients as individuals and has been paramount in influencing and shaping the decisions I make when delivering nursing care, together with planning strategically to manage care. It has also allowed me to recognise, accept and cope with the high level of stress often experienced with working on a demanding, acute medical ward. It has allowed me to receive and offer support to my colleagues by developing a good therapeutic relationship within the nursing team.

Conclusion

In both clinical areas the world consisted of two polarities. One was the concept of chaos and unpredictability, where nothing was secure, nothing was assumed and nothing was assured. At the other pole lay the perhaps false assuredness of the medical model, and its acceptance of the world of science. The nurses in both clinical areas had to deal with people – people who came in all shapes and sizes, with all sorts of experiences, views and attitudes, beliefs and values. This compounded the notion of chaos and the unpredictability of the nursing world. The nurses had to manoeuvre this world of chaos whilst reacting to the scientific quest of medicine to diagnose.

The reductionist simplicity of the medical model could reduce the person to sign and symptom which then portrayed a diagnosis and treatment plan, which in turn offered something of a raft in this world of chaos. The nurses in both clinical areas sometimes had to get on the raft, and sometimes had to swim in the uncharted seas of human experience and behaviour. In other words the nurses had the choice of either practising patient-focused care, and all that that entailed, or reducing their activity quite dramatically to that of doing specific tasks and routines. The reflective group was helping them better chart those seas and not to depend so on that medical raft which seemed somewhat frail and unsuited for the job. In charting these seas though, the nurses had to deal with a number of moral dilemmas and predicaments; they somehow had to find a new understanding of their purpose but the searching for this purpose and identity provided real insecurity, fear, anger, confusion and self-doubt. As they charted these seas they always knew that the organisational premise was that nurses should not worry about making decisions with regard to patient care. It was the doctors who did the thinking and provided the answers. Yet the nurses' experiences told them the doctors often did not have the answers to the questions that the patients asked, therefore there seemed to be a puzzle over the control of nursing in both clinical areas.

Both clinical areas aim to provide patient centred care, both believed that the patient should negotiate the type of nursing that they desired, yet often the traditional task allocation of patient care, of doing the work, getting the jobs done, took precedence over the desire for patient centred care. This servicing of the hospital system and the medical profession would complicate matters, because in both clinical areas nurses would be left with a feeling of guilt and failure, so they sought compromise and rationalisation. They would offer choice, but reflective analysis proved that the choice was somewhat fickle and really consisted of persuasion to do what the nurse or the doctor wanted the patient to do.

There was often a sense of tokenism to achieving patient centred care, but there was also often a sense of great personal development and achievement by the teams when it was achieved, in particular when nurses took the lead with patients over their care, when all others in health care had divorced themselves from certain scenarios. In these cases the phenomenon of 'active' nursing became the norm. They are also grappling with the fact that some patients/people do not actually need nurses, so in both clinical areas there is a growing awareness that the construction of the sickness/illness/hospital provision is not really necessarily beneficial to patient care and some patients would be better cared for at home.

Perhaps, the most important consequence of doing the reflective work with me has been that in both clinical areas the concept of what constitutes health and need has been clarified. As already stated, nurses do not work with illness and diagnostic signs of symptoms, they work with people. Kleinman (1981) stated that the purpose of nursing is to work with the person who is experiencing the illness. The nurse should be able to understand how the illness causes the individual to alter their perceptions of themselves, of their life, of their family, perhaps even of their very existence. This needs careful consideration, nurturing and reflection by the nurse.

In both areas, management support was real and encouraging to the activity. That is, time and space were provided to do the work, 'time-back' existed for those who came in their own time. However, it could be suggested that in the medical ward's case the hospital organisation is somewhat anxious about the prospects of change, but they do seek to harness the change that has taken place and incorporate it into a multi-professional development unit. The outcome of such a venture has yet to be seen.

The reflective process has enabled the nurses to talk with greater ease with each other about their nursing values, beliefs and views and to not feel ashamed or inexpert about sharing their experiences of working with people and their many foibles. The inductive approach to their learning had secured greater relevance to how they thought of themselves, as nurses, and the work that they did. This proved to be a more powerful medium of learning than the conventional didactic approach. As for me, would I change the process and structure of reflection? No, I would not. I feel the structure and process enables such a rich insight to be gained that I look forward to doing further work with these colleagues and I am seeking new areas in order to repeat the activity. I thank my colleagues wholeheartedly.

References

Allen, D. (1985) Nursing research and social control: alternative models of science that emphasise understanding and emancipation. *Image: Journal of Nursing Scholarship*, **XVII**(2), 58–64.

Buckenham, J.E. & McGrath, G. (1983) *The Social Reality of Nursing*. Health Science Press, Sydney.

Emden, C. (1991) Become a reflective practitioner. In *Toward a Discipline of Nursing* (eds G. Gray & R. Pratt). Churchill Livingstone, Melbourne.

Fay, B. (1987) *Critical Social Science*. Polity Press, Cambridge.

Freeman, R. (1996) *How to become a Nursing Development Unit: a guide*. Kings Fund Nursing development programme. Kings Fund, London.

Heron, J. (1992) *Feeling and Personhood Psychology in Another Key*. Sage Publications, London.

Kleinman, A. (1981) The failure of western medicine. In *The Nation's Health* (eds P.R. Lee & I. Red) pp. 18–20. Boyd & Frazer Pub Co., San Francisco.

Lawler, J. (1991) *Behind the Screens. Nursing, Somology and the Problem of the Body*. Churchill Livingstone, Melbourne.

Nightingale, F. (1859) *Notes on Nursing: Nursing What it is and is not*. Wadman, Edinburgh.

Reason, P. & Rowan, J. (1981) On making sense. *Human Inquiry: a Sourcebook of New Paradigm Research*. Wiley, Chichester.

Reason, P. (1988) Human inquiry in action. *Developments in new Paradigm Research*. Sage Publications, London.

Rogers, C. (1970) *Carl Rogers on Encounter Groups*. Harper & Row Pubs. Inc., New York.

Salvage, J. (1984) *The Politics of Nursing*. Heinemann Nursing, London.

Schön, D. (1987) *Educating the Reflective Practitioner*. Jossey-Bass, San Francisco.

Thompson, J.L. (1985) Practical discourse in nursing: going beyond empiricism and historicism. *Advances in Nursing Science*, **4**(4), 59–71.

Van Manen, M. (1990) Researching lived experience. *Human Science for an Action Sensitive Pedagogy*. Althouse Press, Alberta Canada.

Chapter 11

Locating a Phenomenological Perspective of Reflective Nursing and Midwifery Practice by Contrasting Interpretive and Critical Reflection

Bev Taylor

Introduction

In Australian universities the teachers of nursing and midwifery courses have tended to adopt reflective practitioner concepts and strategies (Executive Summary 1994, p. 17). This tendency can be traced to 1988, when educationalists offering postgraduate courses in education to nurses, introduced some principles of critical theory and connected them to reflective practice. The practical evidence of this trend was the emergence of a certain kind of language in nursing curricula and practice, which included words such as reflection and emancipation, and the appearance on the wards and nursing units of exercise books that were used as journals and reflective logs.

Reflective practice was introduced to nurses and midwives in a way which encouraged them to reflect on and in their practice worlds, and to develop ways of changing them (Schön 1983, 1987; Carr & Kemmis 1984; Boud *et al.* 1985; Smyth 1986). This intention carried with it a strong critical theory flavour derived from Marxist politics, which encouraged nurses and midwives to assess the status quo to find the constraining factors within it. Having done this, they were exhorted to find strategies for freeing themselves from these forces, to be liberated to more empowered and effective practice (Habermas 1972; Bernstein 1978; Giroux 1983).

This chapter will focus on phenomenology as an influence in interpretive reflection, by contrasting it with critical reflection, which has been informed by critical theory. In order to differentiate between interpretive and critical reflection, three broad categories of nursing and midwifery knowledge will be described. Following this, three phenomenological concepts will be discussed and their connections to reflective practice, and how reflective processes influenced by phenomenology and critical theory are different from one another. The chapter will conclude by pointing to the relative merit of both approaches as they apply to reflective practice for nurses and midwives.

Three broad categories of nursing and midwifery knowledge (empirical, interpretive, critical)

The basic reason for reflection is to make sense of experience. It is a short step from that assumption to infer that the sense that comes out of reflection is a kind of knowledge which can be recalled and used on other occasions. This is where it gets tricky, because knowledge generation and validation is a very wide and deep area of human interest. For a long time, people have searched for the meaning in life, and their explorations are recorded in the history of ideas, as put forward by philosophers (Palmer 1988). Philosophers are interested in the two main big questions about human life: 'What count as human knowledge?' and 'What is the experience of existence?'. The first question is about epistemology (knowledge generation and validation) and the second question is about ontology (the meaning of the existence of people and things).

A way to make a path through the philosophical maze is to think of three very broad and arbitrary categories of knowledge which apply to nursing, and these can be described as empirical, interpretive and critical. It is important to consider these categories as ways of creating a tidy framework on which to hang certain broad principles. Do not be seduced into thinking that the three forms of knowledge are the only ways of thinking about kinds of knowledge. There are many. Also, do not be fooled into thinking that these three forms of knowledge are dramatically opposed. They share common features. For example, all three approaches can use deductive and inductive thinking, and they require 'scientific' research designs in the sense that they must show that they are systematic and rigorous. Even so, thinking about three forms of knowledge can be useful. A different approach to the task of making a track through the kinds of human knowledge could result in becoming lost in the detail, and that would be tantamount to going on a trek in a strange place without map and compass.

At the outset it may also be helpful to clear up some important terms that form the structure of the chapter. Research is mentioned often in this chapter as a formal means of generating and validating knowledge. Reflection is also mentioned as a means of doing the same, but it may be more informal in that it may not need to be related to an actual research project and conform to the standard requirements for research proposals. Knowledge is generated through research and reflection. In this chapter, differentiation will be made between interpretive knowledge which may be informed by phenomenological perspectives of reflective practice, and critical knowledge which may be informed by critical theory perspectives of reflective practice. The reason for this approach is that the language of reflective practice has been typically of a critical reflective flavour, and to date little differentiation has been made between the origins, nature and effects of interpretive and critical reflection.

Empirical knowledge

Empirical knowledge is that which is generated and tested through 'the scientific method' of research. When the strict conditions of the scientific method are fulfilled, the empirical knowledge that results is considered to be absolute, which means it claims to be complete, perfect and free from limitations. Empirical knowledge is concerned with making cause and effect links, and it is created through deductive thinking processes which move systematically from broad to focused inferences. To generate knowledge through research, questions are hypothesised as likely or unlikely outcomes, ideas are tested through observation and analysis, and numbers are used to convey information as mathematical relationships.

To be able to claim that knowledge is faithful and true, research conditions require validity through the control of variables. This means that the project is designed carefully to ensure that the thing being tested is the thing intended, and that related and unexpected things are not tested by accident or by poor planning. In order to show that knowledge is real and true the reliability of it is determined through test and retest. Findings are quantified in numbers, which need to be significant statistically, so that they can be predictive and claim to be generalisable. This gives some confidence that the result is truthful, real, and trust-worthy and not just happening by chance.

Methods for collecting empirical data include controlled trials, experiments, surveys and questionnaires. To banish emotionality and personal prejudice in the collecting and analysing of data, objectivity is important to gain knowledge which is free of human distortions. To make projects manageable and systematic, problem areas for research are reduced to their smallest parts.

The outcomes of this method for the generation of empirical knowledge include description of what is, prediction for what might be, and change through new knowledge discoveries (Taylor 1995). The success of empirical knowledge is evident in nursing and midwifery through the continued and updated support of medical advances and the constant evolution of newer and safer technical nursing and midwifery procedures.

Interpretive and critical knowledge

The interpretive and critical categories differ from the empirical knowledge form, and they differ from each other. However, interpretive and critical categories of knowledge have more features in common than they have dissimilarities, so will be considered together in this section, before their major differences are emphasised.

Interpretive and critical categories feature knowledge which is relative, and which is seen to be centred in the people and their place, time and conditions. Inductive thinking is used which starts from the specific instance and moves to the general pattern of combined instances, so that it grows from 'the ground up' to make larger statements about the nature of the thing being investigated. Rather than starting with a statement of hypothesis of what may or may not be found, interpretive and critical knowledge uses a research approach which leaves open the possible outcomes and begins typically with a statement of the area of interest.

The measures for ensuring validity involve asking the participants to confirm that interpretations are represented faithfully and clearly for them by the researcher. Reliability is often not an issue, based on the idea that knowledge is relative and that it is dependent on all the features of the people, place, time and other circumstances of the context. This means that it is highly unlikely that projects could be repeated in exactly the same way, and that the people involved would give exactly the same answers as they did previously.

People are valued as sources of information, and their expressions of subjectivity are acknowledged as being integral to the meaning that comes out of the research. Rather than requiring results to be statistically significant, interpretive and critical research approaches make no claims to generate knowledge that can be relied on as absolute. Instead, there is acknowledgment that people and things may change according to their circumstances, so it is inappropriate to generalise research findings to a wider group of people or things being studied. This means that research topics can be explored by a variety of means, such as interviews, participant observation and storytelling, and that words can be used as the basis for analysis.

Although interpretive and critical categories of knowledge have assumptions in common about the relative context-dependent and subjective nature of knowledge, they have some major differences. The differences lie in the intentions for, and the processes of, knowledge generation and validation. All three categories can bring about change through the generation of new knowledge. It is the way it is done that differs. For example, new empirical knowledge generated through the scientific method can shift and change human thought about the facts known and applied to human and natural phenomena.

Change may also occur as a result of the generation of interpretive and critical knowledge. When new knowledge is generated through interpretive methods people may raise their awareness of something and make adaptations in their perceptions and/or actions to accommodate the new insights. Research approaches that create interpretive knowledge include grounded theory, phenomenology, historical research and ethnography. Interpretive enquiry may include some participation of the people involved, but the collaboration between researcher and researched may be minimal to moderate and participants are not regarded generally as co-researchers with 'ownership' of the project.

In critical knowledge the 'up front' intention is to bring about change, therefore people with the problems get together to work through ways of solving them. Processes used usually involve a moderate to high degree of participation and collaboration of the people involved, who are valued as co-researchers. Research approaches that create critical knowledge to bring about change intentionally include action research, feminist research, interpretive interactionism and critical ethnography.

The reason for this brief sojourn into categories of knowledge is to differentiate between major paradigms, or world views, of possible epistemological categories. In a general sense, interpretive reflection uses some epistemological assumptions of phenomenology, and critical reflection uses some assumptions of critical theory. Put another way, phenomenology lies in the interpretive paradigm or world view of epistemology. Structured reflection creates interpretive knowledge for generating meaning and change through raised awareness. Critical theory lies in the critical paradigm. Structured reflection creates critical knowledge for providing a radical critique of the status quo to bring about intentional and positive social and political change.

This brings us back to the introduction to this section, in order to reiterate and extend some ideas about knowledge and reflection. The practical outcome of reflection is making sense of things, thereby generating new or amended knowledge that may have the potential for change. Empirical, interpretive and critical knowledge may be generated through reflection. The two main kinds of reflection in nursing and midwifery practice are interpretive and critical. Interpretive reflection informed by some phenomenological assumptions may generate interpretive knowledge. Critical reflection informed by critical theory may generate critical knowledge.

Principles underlying reflective nursing and midwifery practice

In essence, reflective practice is the systematic and thoughtful means by which practitioners can make sense of their practice as they go about their daily work. The need for reflection-in-action as it happens, and reflection-on-action after the event, is built on the supposition that practitioners know more than they realise and they need ways of bringing that knowledge to their realisation (Schön 1983). In Australia there seems to be general acceptance that reflective practice is appropriate and desirable for nurses and midwives. The importance of reflective practice has been written into a national document as necessary 'for the improvement of the quality of teaching in nursing in higher education' (Executive Summary 1994, p. 17).

Another underlying principle of reflective practice is that practitioners have a tendency to take their knowledge and skills for granted, and when talking about their mode of employment they tend to preface their comments with, 'I'm just a nurse/midwife'. Blumberg (1990, p. 236) argued that practitioners need 'to change how they think about their work', in that they need to value themselves as practitioners and the knowledge and skills of their day to day practice.

Unfortunately, systematic and purposeful reflection is not necessarily 'second nature' to people. Schön (1987) argued that practitioners need coaching to deal with practice problems. Other writers agree that coaching is necessary and that it promotes collaborative knowing (Greenwood 1993; Conway 1994). Coaching in reflective processes also encourages co-operative communication between the instructor and participants (Belenky *et al.* 1986). Newell (1992) and Von Wright (1992) also claim that education is needed in the art of reflection. Emphasising the need for purposeful and systematic reflection, Newell (1992) argued that mentors and support persons need time in training and support themselves, in order to be of service to others in coaching them in reflective skills. In the case of practitioners of mature age, however, it might be expected that without too much effort adults can build on their life experiences to make sense out of what happens at work (Knowles 1980). Therefore, a principle underlying reflective practice for nurses and midwives is that, with adequate coaching, they will be able to achieve systematic and purposeful reflection.

There are various means by which practitioners may undertake reflective practice. Methods for reflection include journal writing, metaphor analysis, storytelling and portfolio development (Caffarella & Barnett 1994). Schön (1987) suggested the use of reflective diaries for personal reflections. Nurses and midwives have a rich oral tradition and they have many stories to tell. Therefore, personal reflections in diaries or on audio tape, about interesting and possibly disturbing events, may be a favoured means of assisting reflection.

As reflective practice may be undertaken in many ways, the choice of the kind of reflection may be determined to some extent by the kind of knowledge that people are seeking to generate in and through their practice. If practitioners are intending to increase their understanding of points of interest in their practice, they might lean towards phenomenologically informed reflective assumptions and strategies. The types of questions that nurses and midwives could pose when engaging in interpretive reflection might include: 'What is happening here?', 'What is the nature of. . . ?', 'What is the experience of. . . ?'.

If practitioners are intending to change the constraining nature and effects of political, economic, cultural, social and historical elements in their practice, they might prefer approaches informed by critical theory as a basis for their reflective assumptions and strategies. The types of questions that nurses and midwives could pose when engaging in critical reflection might include: 'What is happening here?', 'What factors have made it this way. . . ?', 'How might this be different. . . ?'.

Phenomenological influences in interpretive reflection

Historically, phenomenology emerged around the turn of the twentieth century. Up until the seventeenth century, philosophical thought included some musings about natural elements, such as air, fire, water and earth, as well as gods and God. From that time, there was a swing towards needing to prove things were truthful by the application of scientific means, and this tradition has lasted strongly to the present time as emprico-analytical knowledge. However, within the 90+ years of the twentieth century, there have been critiques of the dominant world view of science.

The turning point in epistemology came when some philosophers started to argue that the scientific method, described in this chapter as empirical knowledge, was not sufficient in human enquiry. They claimed that it did not explain and describe things about human life that relate to a sense of self (subjectivity) and awareness of inner and outer experiences (consciousness). Philosophers such as Edmund Husserl (1960, 1964), and Martin Heidegger (1962 trans.) began to talk and write about the importance of using human subjectivity to understand human knowing and existence. In doing this, they readmitted effectively into philosophy, open and active discussions about subjectivity and consciousness, that had been disbanded, to a great extent, by the prominence of empirico-analytic methods of knowledge generation and validation.

Although at least six types of phenomenology have been described (Speigelberg 1970), it is possible to speak generally of phenomenology. Phenomenology acknowledges and values the meanings people give to their own existence. The catch-cry of phenomenology from the time of Husserl has been: 'To the things!' (*Zu den Sachen*), meaning that its prime intent is to discover, explore and describe things as they are as 'uncensored phenomena' (Spiegelberg 1970, p. 21), as they are immediately given. This means that everything is open to enquiry and that enquiry is directed at finding the essential nature of the thing (phenomenon) of interest.

Phenomenology allows philosophers and researchers to explore the nature of something from a close and intense study of it as a thing of interest. Phenomenological enquiry has been, and continues to be, immense and intense (Husserl 1960 trans, 1964 trans, 1965 trans, 1970, 1980 trans; Heidegger 1962; Merleau-Ponty 1962, 1967; Kockelmans 1967; Spiegelberg 1970, 1975, 1976; Zaner 1970, 1971; Gadamer 1975, 1976; Krell 1977; Scheiermacher 1977 trans; Langveld 1978; Van Manen 1978–79, 1984; Hekman 1986; Palmer 1988; Dreyfus 1991). Given that nurses and midwives may not aspire to be either philosophers or researchers, a short-cut way of thinking about phenomenology is to consider selected basic concepts which underlie much of its theoretical content. Three useful concepts will be addressed here: lived experience, context and subjectivity.

Lived experience

Some nurses (Gulino 1982; Oiler 1982, 1986; Aamodt 1983; Parse *et al.* 1985; Drew 1986; Reiman, 1986; McPherson 1987; Bergum 1989; Forrest

1989; Kretlow 1989–1990) claim that phenomenology is mainly about understanding lived experience, which means it is about knowing what it is like to live a life in a particular time, place and set of circumstances. People live out their lives on a day to day basis in ways that are relatively unique and individualistic, and the level of conscious awareness of their existence may vary between people. Dilthey (1985 trans.) suggested that lived experience is awareness of life without thinking about it, a pre-reflexive consciousness of life. He explained that:

> 'lived experience does not confront me as something perceived or represented; it is not given to me, but the reality of the lived experi-ence is there-for-me because I have reflexive awareness of it, because I possess it immediately as belonging to me in some sense. Only in thought does it become objective.' (p. 223)

Reflection is the key to making sense of human existence, because lived experiences accumulate and gather interpretive significance as they are remembered. By thinking about what has happened and is happening to themselves, to others and to other things of interest, people get a sense of finding some meaning which is relevant to themselves and may be helpful for others with whom it resonates. This concept of lived experience fits very well with the principles of reflective practice, and it shows quite clearly the relevance of phenomenology in deciding on questions that promote interpretive reflection.

The concept of lived experience refers to how it is to live a life in regard to being someone or something unique. This infers that every human has lived experiences. Dogs, cats, trees, and all other living things also have lived experiences, but they may be relatively unable to communicate them to a human, so the concept of lived experience is best pondered in relation to human experiences. This is one of the challenges of certain kinds of phenomenology: to arrive at the meaning of lived human experiences and put them out in the public arena for others to contemplate.

Gadamer (1976) acknowledged the value of lived experience of peo-ple, especially in respect to its potential to join together universal and personal aspects of their worlds. This basically means that he thought that a lot could be learned about the wider stage of life, through understanding the existence of the individual actors. Through living out a day to day existence, he claimed that people were able potentially to locate phenomena that were questionable within the so-called objective world. In other words, he considered that a personal experience of day to day life was instructive for locating and understanding bigger and broader things out there and distant from the day to day concerns of personal life.

Context

Context is another phenomenologically informed principle of interpretive reflection. Context means all of the features of the time and place in which people find themselves, and in which they locate their descriptions of things and people in their lives. People live their daily lives in the moment, yet they also remain connected to their past and hopeful of their future (Heidegger 1962). Being human and living a life suggests some passage of time and some continuity in daily inter-personal relationships and events. People cannot help but be placed and involved in their particular time and place situations. The familiarity of the context provides relative security for daily activity, and novel situations may be managed with reference to like situations of which people have had previous experience.

Context sets the scene for the interpretation of lived experience, because people are always situated in time and space. In agreement with the definition of lived experience given by Dilthey (1985), Dreyfus (1979, in Benner & Wrubel 1989, p. 83) claimed that 'we are able to move around in the everyday world because our understanding is always situated and our actions are typically only as orderly as the situation demands'. The familiarity of the context provides relative security for daily activity. Novel situations may be managed with reference to like situations of which people have had previous experience. This seems true of nursing and midwifery practice. Practitioners are very familiar with the work setting and circumstances and thus they feel ready for what may transpire as part of the work day. Practitioners seem to know what to do and how to do it in certain unforeseen circumstances.

Contextually appropriate understandings and actions have been described by Benner & Wrubel (1989, p. 412), who refer to 'situation,' as the 'the relevant concerns, issues, information, constraints, and resour-ces at a given span of time or place as experienced by particular persons'. In applying this principle to healthcare settings, practitioners and clients make sense of their situations 'in terms of their own personal concerns, background meanings, temporality, habitual, cultural bodies, emotions and reflective thoughts' (p. 82). Translated into language of a more digestible nature, this means that nurses and clients work out what to do and how to do it in any situation by making personal applications to their own life issues, worries and stories, and to their sense of time, habits and favoured rituals and patterns of behaviour in various groups. They also pay attention to how they feel and what sense they make from it based on experience. All of these things happen in an instant. This shows sophistication in rapid thinking and acting, which is possible from being the inhabitant of a physical body with all its past, present and future potential.

Subjectivity

Subjectivity refers to the individual's sensing of inner and external things. Subjective or personal knowledge does not make a universal claim to be true for everyone and for all things in all times and places, rather it refers to personal experiences and personal truths that may or may not be like other people's subjective experiences and truths. In the social world of daily life, humans take account of one another's sense of self and they share their experiences and truths through what is referred to as 'intersubjectivity'. In interpretive research such as phenomenology, attempts are made to understand various relationships between people, by taking account of relationships between people as they are expressed by them.

People exist in social contexts, in communication with other people's time and space circumstances. In the social world of daily life, humans take account of one another and share their experiences and truths in an intersubjective dialogue. Nursing and midwifery occur in social contexts in which intersubjective meanings are generated. Nurses and midwives cannot help but interpret their work experiences from their respective intersubjective viewpoints. They know that:

> 'the best nursing [and midwifery] practitioners understand the differences and relationships among health, illness and disease. This understanding leads nurses [and midwives] to seek the patient's story in formal and informal nursing histories, because they know that every illness has a story – plans that are threatened or thwarted, relationships are disturbed, and symptoms become laden with meaning depending on what else is happening in the person's life...'
> (Benner & Wrubel 1989, p.9)

Interpretive reflection informed by the phenomenological concepts of lived experience, context and subjectivity generates knowledge that is personal and practical. Interpretive knowledge emerges from the perspectives of the actual people who are engaged actively in their worlds. Interpretive reflection values what people feel and think. No questions are raised about the 'truthfulness' of the accounts, as faith is placed in the veracity of the accounts. Nor are measures taken to ensure objectivity, because subjective experience is acknowledged as being instructive for bigger and wider issues beyond personal accounts. These assumptions are in keeping with the phenomenological concepts of lived experience, context and subjectivity. Missing from these phenomenological concepts, however, are ideas of critique and political intention. These ideas feature in critical reflection informed by critical theory.

Critical theory influences in critical reflection

Critical theory and theorising seeks to look into what is promoted as the status quo of various repressive social contexts, to discover and expose the forces that maintain them for their particular advantages. This means that it looks at the way things are and asks how they might be different and better for the majority of people, not just the privileged few. As human social constructions, knowledge and social existence represent identifiable human interests (Habermas 1972). As a critical theorist, Habermas argued that human knowledge could be categorised as technical (empirical knowledge), practical (interpretive knowledge) and emancipatory (critical knowledge). These kinds of knowledge relate to people's vested interests in their lives.

Another principle underlying critical theory is that knowledge serves certain purposes which may be seen as 'immutable' and 'inevitable', thereby maintaining as unquestioned the advantages of the powerful elite they favour. In less turgid language, this sentence translates in the following way. One of the purposes knowledge serves is to maintain the influence of powerful people and regimes, and keep other people 'down'. The subordination is so effective that the less powerful people think that the situation cannot be changed and that the powerful forces are appropriate and acceptable, even though they are actually repressive to them in many ways.

The emancipatory critique of critical theory relies on systematic reflection and promises freedom from the distorted understandings, communication and activities of pre-existing social structures, giving possibilities for new ways of being and acting within them (Bernstein 1978, 1983). In nursing and midwifery, this relates to relationships of nurses and midwives with other workers and among themselves, within the context of specific healthcare settings, and within the larger national system. This might mean, for example, that through systematic reflection and critique, nurses and midwives will learn to be free from their own perceptions that their subservient role relationships with doctors and health administrators are unchanging and inevitable. Instead of claiming that they are unable to change the status quo by saying, 'It has always been this way', or 'That's the way it is', nurses and midwives may learn to ask, 'How could this be different and better for me and for my colleagues?'

The promises of critical theory that are either implied or made explicit in reflective practitioner processes relate to the nature of critical theory as a philosophical position and as a process of theorising (Giroux 1983). Critical theory offers freedom. Change for the better is the main interest of critical reflection. The change may mean freedom from people's previous perceptions of themselves and their circumstances, and freedom to change to something that is better for them. This means that there is a liberatory intent in using radical critiques to transform the existing restrictive social order and conditions within the status quo into those that are based and enacted on the principles of equality, freedom and justice. The idea is to question, critique and systematically topple the dominant forces that prevent the equitable distribution of money, knowledge, opportunities and power.

Comparing and valuing interpretive and critical reflection

A phenomenological perspective of reflection will offer nurses and midwives the potential for creating interpretive knowledge which is

informative about the meaning of lived experience, context and subjectivity. It will also offer potential for change, based on raised awareness of the nature of a wide range of matters pertaining to nursing and
midwifery. What interpretive reflection will not offer is the kind of
knowledge which will provide a systematic critique of the constraining
forces and influences within the status quo of nurses' and midwives'
work settings. A phenomenological perspective in reflective processes
will also not offer a political imagination which analyses people in their
situations in terms of their propensity to seek their own advantage and
power.

For some time now in nursing and midwifery (Speedy 1987, 1988;
Pearson, 1988, 1989; Holmes 1990, 1992; Gray & Pratt 1991; Lawler 1991;
Lumby 1991) and allied literature (Carr & Kemmis 1984; Smyth 1986),
the critique of interpretive knowledge in general is that it fails to move
beyond description of meaning to something more important, and that it
is social and political change. This is an acceptable critique if it is reasonable to contrast the assumptions of one paradigm of knowledge
against those of another. It is also an acceptable critique if one can claim
successfully that one form of knowledge is more preferred, valid and
useful than another.

The assumptions of phenomenology and critical theory differ as to the
intentions, processes and outcomes of knowledge. It is inevitable that
phenomenology will continue to be criticised for not going far enough to
address social and political issues in nursing and midwifery, even
though that is not its prime intention. There is room in nursing and
midwifery theory and practice for multiple perspectives of knowledge.
There is room for various kinds of interpretive knowledge generally and
knowledge derived from phenomenological perspectives specifically. It
follows then that there is room for phenomenological perspectives of
reflective practice. Not all situations in nursing and midwifery are about
intentional change. There is still much that needs to be understood about
the nature and effects of nursing and midwifery practice. With fuller and
clearer description of the phenomena of interest to nursing and midwifery practice, new ideas may surface and there may be greater insights
into the nature and effects of the work. With this may come enhanced
potential for positive change.

With respect to the inferred superiority of one from of knowledge over
another in terms of its preference, validity and usefulness, this matter
has been addressed previously and capably by Carper (1978) and Chinn
& Kramer (1991). These American nurses claim that there are many
ways of knowing, that each of these ways has merit and usefulness, and
that there is no hierarchy in their importance (Carper 1978). For these
women, knowledge includes empirical, personal, aesthetic and ethical
forms. Respectively, these ways of knowing are concerned basically with
scientifically observed, analysed and validated facts, personal insights,
knowledge of the beautiful, and moral judgements. Carper also made
the point that these ways of knowing need to be balanced and inte-

grated. This argument was taken up by Chinn & Kramer (1991), who claimed that too much reliance on one way of thinking and knowing about things can cause distortions. For example, too much empirical knowledge may result in the tendency to control and manipulate, too much personal knowledge may result in isolation and self-distortion, too much aesthetics may result in prejudice and bigotry, and too much ethical knowledge may result in rigid doctrine and insensitivity to others (Chinn & Kramer 1991).

Using this reasoning it seems fairly appropriate to infer that one kind of knowledge is equal to any other. Balance is important in the kinds of knowledge generated and verified in research and reflection, to try to ensure that ideas, descriptions and explanations have the best chance of being well rounded and comprehensive. Knowledge itself is not at fault for considering itself superior; rather it is human interpretation which puts it in that position. Knowledge exists for all sorts of purposes and the means people use to find it will determine to some extent the way it looks and the purposes it serves. In other words, if nurses or midwives are trying to generate meaning and potential change in their practice through raised awareness of new insights, interpretive reflection may be the most appropriate approach. If nurses or midwives are trying to address inequities and problems in work settings, relationships and circumstances, critical reflection may be of more use to them.

Conclusion

Nurses and midwives engaged in daily practice have the advantage of living their practice, in that they have opportunities to look at their practice to learn from it. When nurses reflect on what they do, they can make sense of their practice, and imagine and/or bring about changes (Street 1991; Cox *et al.* 1991). The kinds of changes they desire might direct the kind of reflection they use.

Interpretive knowledge is useful and it has a place in the balanced and integrated whole of human knowledge. This chapter attempted to reinforce that claim by locating phenomenology within three broad epistemological categories, and contrasting its perceived strengths and limitations with that of critical theory. All kinds of knowledge can be generated through reflection. Nurses and midwives can benefit from a range of reflective processes which have been informed by assumptions about the way knowledge is produced and proven. The first questions to ask in making a choice between interpretive and critical reflection are: 'What do I want to know through reflection?', 'Why do I want to know it?' and 'What questions will stimulate and guide my reflections and lead me to the answers I am seeking?'.

If nurses and midwives want to better understand themselves, other people and other things, they would be well advised to use a form of interpretive reflection. Interpretive reflection was discussed as processes and questions which may be informed by phenomenological assumptions, and generate a kind of descriptive knowledge which is informative for human enquiry. Critical reflection was discussed as that which had higher possibilities of creating knowledge that could bring about change, because some assumptions of critical theory underlying it are geared towards intentional social and political improvements in the status quo.

The approach taken in this chapter was to situate phenomenology in some broad categories of knowledge, in order to explain the usefulness of applying certain phenomenological perspectives to reflective practice for nurses and midwives.

References

Aamodt, A.M. (1983) Problems in doing nursing research: developing a criteria for evaluating qualitative research. *Western Journal of Nursing Research*, 5, 398–402.

Belenky, M., Clinchy, B., Goldberger, N. & Tarule, J. (1986) *Women's Ways of Knowing*. Basic Books, New York.

Benner, P. & Wrubel, J. (1989) *The Primary of Caring: Stress and Coping in Health and Illness*. Addison-Wesley, Menlo Park.

Bergum, V. (1989) Being a phenomenological researcher. In *Qualitative Nursing Research: A Contemporary Dialogue* (ed. J.M. Morse). Aspen, Maryland.

Bernstein, R.J. (1978) *The Restructuring of Social and Political Theory*. University of Pennsylvannia Press, Philadelphia.

Bernstein, R.J. (1983) *Beyond Objectivism and Relativism: Science, Hermeneutics and Praxis*. University of Pennsylvannia Press, Philadelphia.

Blumberg, A. (1990) Toward a scholarship of practice. *Journal of Curriculum and Supervision*. **5**(3) 236–43.

Boud, D., Keogh, R. & Walker, D. (1985) *Reflection: Turning Experience into Learning*. Kogan Page, London.

Carper, B.A. (1978) Fundamental patterns of knowing in nursing. *Advances in Nursing Science*, 1, 13–23.

Carr, W. & Kemmis, S. (1984) *Becoming Critical: Knowing Through Action Research*. Deakin University Press, Victoria.

Caffarella, R. & Barnett, B. (1994) Characteristics of adult learners and foundations of experiential learning. *New Directions for Adult and Continuing Education*, number 62, summer. Jossey Bass, San Francisco.

Chinn, P.L. & Kramer, M.K. (1991) *Theory and Nursing: A Systematic Approach*, 3rd edn. Mosby Year Book, St Louis.

Conway, J. (1994) Reflection, the art and science of nursing and the theory-practice gap. *British Journal of Nursing*, 393, 114–18.

Cox, H. Hickson, P. & Taylor, B.J. (1991) Exploring reflection: knowing and constructing the practice of nursing. In *Towards a Discipline of Nursing* (eds G. Gray & R. Pratt), pp. 373–89. Churchill Livingstone, London.

Dilthey, W. (1985) *Poetry and Experience. Selected Works*, vol V. Princeton University Press, New Jersey.

Drew, N. (1986) Exclusion and confirmation: a phenomenology of patients' experiences with caregivers. *Image: Journal of Nursing Scholarship*, **18**(2), 39–43.

Dreyfus, H.L. (1991) *Being-In-The World: A Commentary on Heidegger's Being and Time*. Division 1, The MIT Press, Cambridge, MA.

Executive Summary (1994) *Nursing education in Australian universities*. Report of the National Review of Nurse Education in the Higher Education Sector 1994 and Beyond. Australian Government Publishing service, Canberra.

Forrest, D. (1989) The experience of caring. *Journal of Advanced Nursing*, 14, 815–23.

Gadamer, H-G. (1975) *Truth and Method* (ed. & trans. by G. Barden & J. Cumming). Seabury, New York.

Gadamer, H-G. (1976) *The Universality of the Hermeneutical Problem*. Philosophical Hermeneutics, Linge, D E trans. University of California Press, Berkeley.

Giroux, H.A. (1983) *Theory and Resistance in Education: a Pedagaogy for the Opposition*. Bergin & Garvey, South Hadley, Massachusetts.

Gray, G. & Pratt, R. (eds) (1991) *Toward the Discipline of Nursing*. Churchill Livingstone, Sydney.

Greenwood, J. (1993) Reflective practice: a critique of the work of Argyris & Schön. *Journal of Advanced Nursing*, 18, 1183–7.

Gulino, C.K. (1982) Entering the mysterious dimensions of others: an existential approach to nursing care. *Nursing Outlook*, **30**(6) 352–7.

Habermas, J. (1972) *Knowledge and Human Interests*. Heinemann, London.

Heidegger, M. (1962) *Being and Time* (trans. by J. Macquarrie & E. Robinson). Harper & Row, New York.

Hekman, S.J. (1986) *Hermeneutics and the Sociology of Knowledge*. Polity Press, Cambridge.

Holmes, C. (1990) Alternatives to natural science foundations for nursing. *International Journal of Nursing Studies*, **27** (3), 187–98.

Holmes, C. (1992) The drama of nursing. *Journal of Advanced Nursing*, 17, 954–60.

Husserl, E. (1960) *Cartesian Meditations: an Introduction to Phenomenology* (trans. by D. Cairns). Matinus Nijhoff, The Hague.

Husserl, E. (1964) *The Idea of Phenomenology* (trans. by W.P. Alston & G. Nakhnikian). Martinus Nijhoff, The Hague.

Husserl, E. (1965) *Phenomenology and the Crisis of Philosophy* (trans. by Q. Lauer). Harper & Row, New York.

Husserl, E. (1970) *The Crisis of The European Sciences And Transcendental Phenomenology*. Northwestern University Press, Evanston.

Husserl, E. (1980) *Phenomenonology And The Foundations of The Sciences* (trans. by T.E. Klein & W.E. Pohl. Martinus Nijhoff, The Hague.

Knowles, M. (1980) *The Modern Practice of Adult Education: from Pedagogy to Andragogy*, 2nd edn. Cambridge Book Co, New York.

Kockelmans, J. J. (ed) (1967) *Phenomenology: the Philosophy of Edmund Husserl and its Interpretation*. Anchor Books, Doubleday & Company, Garden City, New York.

Krell, D.F. (1977) *Martin Heidegger: Basic Writings*. Harper & Row, New York.

Kretlow, F. (1989-1990) A phenomenological view of illness. *The Australian Journal of Advanced Nursing*, **7**(2), 8–10.

Langveld, M.J. (1978) The stillness of the secret place. *Phenomenology and Pedagogy*, **1**(1), 181–9.

Lawler, J. (1991) In search of an Australian identity. In *Toward the Discipline of Nursing* (eds G. Gray & R. Pratt), pp, 211–27. Churchill Livingstone, Sydney.

Lumby, J (1991) *Nursing: Reflecting on an Evolving Practice*. Deakin University Press, Geelong,

McPherson, P. (1987) The quality of being expressed as doing. *The Australian Journal of Advanced Nursing*, **5**(1) 38–42.

Merleau-Ponty, M. (1962) *Phenomenology of Perception.* Routledge & Kegan Paul, London

Merleau-Ponty, M. (1967) What is Phenomenology? In *Phenomenology: the Philosophy of Edmund Husserl and its Interpretation* (ed. J.J. Kockelmans). Doubleday, New York.

Newell, R. (1992) Anxiety, accuracy and reflection: the limits of professional development. *Journal of Advanced Nursing,* 17, 1326–33.

Oiler, C. (1982) The phenomenological approach in nursing research. *Nursing Research,* **31**(3) 171–81.

Oiler, C. (1986) Phenomenology: the method. In *Nursing Research: A Qualitative Perspective* (eds P. Munhall & C. J. Oiler). Appleton-Century-Crofts, Norwalk.

Palmer, D. (1988) *Looking at Philosophy: The Unbearable Heaviness of Philosophy made Lighter.* Mayfield Publishing Company, California.

Parse, R.R. Coyne, A.B. & Smith, M.J. (1985) *Nursing Research: Qualitative Methods.* Brady, Bowie.

Pearson, A. (1988) *Nursing: from whence to where.* Professorial lecture, Deakin University, Geelong.

Pearson, A (1989) Therapeutic nursing-transforming models and theories in action. In Theories and Models in Nursing (ed. J.A. Akinsanya). *Recent Advances in Nursing,* vol. 24, pp. 123–51 Longman Group, Harlow.

Reiman, D.J. (1986) The essential structure of a caring interaction: doing phenomenology. In *Nursing Research: a Qualitative Perspective* (eds P. Munhall & C.J. Oiler). Appleton-Century-Crofts, Norwalk.

Schön, D.A. (1983) *The Reflective Practitioner: How Practitioners Think in Action.* Basic Books, New York.

Schön, D.A. (1987) *Educating the Reflective Practitioner.* Jossey-Bass, London.

Scheiermacher, F. (1977) *Hermeneutics: The Handwritten Manuscripts* (eds H. Kimmerle h & J. Duke, trans. by Fortsman. J. Scholars Press, Atlanta.

Smyth, W.J. (1986) *The reflective practitioner in nursing education.* Unpublished paper to the Second National Nursing Education Seminar, SACAE, Adelaide.

Speedy, S. (1987) Feminism and the professionalization of nursing. *The Australian Journal of Advanced Nursing,* **4**(2), 20–28.

Speedy, S. (1988) Feminism and nursing: theory to practice. *Shaping Nursing Theory and Practice: The Australian Context.* Department of Nursing, LaTrobe University.

Spiegelberg, H. (1970) On some human uses of phenomenology. In *Phenomenology In Perspective* (ed. F.J. Smith). Martinus Nijhoff, The Hague.

Spiegelberg, H. (1975) *Doing Phenomenology.* Martinus Nijhoff, The Hague.

Speigelberg, H. (1976) *The Phenomenological Movement,* vols 1 & 11. Martinus Nijhoff, The Hague.

Street, A. (1991) *From Image to Action: Reflection in Nursing Practice.* Deakin University Press, Geelong.

Taylor, B, (1995) *Qualitative Research Data: What it Can Offer Women's Health Centres.* Centre for Professional Development, Health Sciences, Southern Cross University, Lismore.

Van Manen, M. (1978–79) An experiment in educational theorising: the Utrecht school. *Interchange* **10**(1), 48–66.

Van Manen, M. (1984) *'Doing' Phenomenological Research And Writing: An Introduction.* Monograph No 7. University of Alberta, Edmonton.

Von Wright, J. (1992) Reflections on reflection. *Learning and Instruction,* 12, 59–68.

Zaner, R. (1970) *The Way Of Phenomenology: Criticism as a Philosophical Discipline.* Pegasus, New York.

Zaner, R. (1971) *The Problem of Embodiment: Some Contributions to a Phenomenology of the Body.* Martinus Nijhoff, The Hague.

Chapter 12
Reflection and Expert Nursing Knowledge

Jane Glaze

Introduction

The development of reflective practice is complex. Many factors influence this process and these are explored in some detail in this chapter. The premise of this work is that critical reflection is central to transformation of practice. It may be helpful to ask what is meant by the term transforming practice and what reflective practice has to do with it. According to the Oxford Dictionary transform is a verb which means 'to make a great change to the appearance or character of, for example the caterpillar is transformed into a butterfly'. It can be seen from the emphasis given to 'great change' that transformation is about more than bringing about change. Implicit to this definition is the notion that what one starts out with bears little or no relationship to the end product. The caterpillar is cumbersome, awkward and earth bound. The butterfly in contrast emerges from its catalyst in all of its glory as a newly formed beautiful creature. It is no longer earth bound, but free to fly where it wills.

Whilst this analogy may not exactly apply to nursing there are areas of commonality. Nursing's history has been typified by adherence to ritual and routine (Bevis 1982), and this can be seen as the caterpillar stage. The analogy also applies in that in some areas such constrained practice has been metamorphasised into critical reflective practice (Conway 1995).

Whilst there is a growing body of literature on reflective practice, particular attention will be paid here to considering the links between transforming practice and reflection.

Reflection as a process for transforming nursing practice

Reflection is defined in many ways, and there is ambiguity in the way the term is used. Some elements of transformation can be found in Donald Schön's work in which reflection-in-action is linked to professional development. Indeed, Schön's theories about practice are

151

transformative. He recognises not only that the problems of practice are often messy and ill defined, but also that these are 'the problems of greatest human concern' (Schön 1987). He presents reflection-in-action as a process whereby the professional 'thinks on her feet', finding the solution to problems through framing and reframing. This appears to be an almost subconscious process whereby theory and practice are synthesised into reflection-in-action. Such attributes are identified as typifying only the practice of experienced expert practitioners (Schön 1983, 1987).

Reflection-on-action which occurs after an event is similar to more traditional, accepted interpretations of reflection (Dewey 1933; Boud *et al.* 1985). However, in terms of practice it is clear that it is reflection-in-action that provides new insights and further dimensions to the traditional acceptance of reflection and links these to professional development. In contrast to Schön's work, reflection is presented by Boud *et al.* (1985) as something so familiar that it tends to be overlooked. These differentiations cause difficulties since it is impossible merely by the use of the term reflection to know exactly in what sense the term is being used.

Yet other definitions go beyond simple problem solving approaches and include acknowledgement of a critical process (Carr & Kemmis 1986) allied to retrospection (FEU 1981; Grudy 1982 cited by Boud *et al.* 1985). Perhaps the most challenging for nursing is the critical science perspective. The work of the Frankfurt School of Social Research, and of Habermas in particular, is cited as having:

'inspired a critical science concept of reflection as self-determination. Reflection is viewed as a process of becoming aware of one's context, of the influence of societal and ideological constraints on previously taken-for-granted practices.' (Calderhead 1989)

It can be seen that reflection is used here to describe a liberating and empowering process. It is about developing self-awareness and self-knowledge. Also it requires practitioners to develop a critical element to their thinking:

'... one must become critically conscious of how an ideology reflects and distorts moral, social and political reality and what material and psychological factors influence and sustain the false consciousness which it represents – especially reified powers of domination.' (Mezirow 1981, p. 6)

This ability to become critically conscious is far removed from simply examining an event to see what should be done differently. There is an implicit political dimension, linked to critical awareness, which enables assumptions inherent in ideologies to be challenged. This has been presented by Freire (1970) as conscientisation. This critical perspective of reflection differs considerably from other presentations on the topic (Boud *et al.* 1985; Schön 1983, 1987). It offers an approach to reflection and nursing practice which none of the other theorists present. The assumption within emancipatory theory is that challenging of ideologies is possible. While this is desirable there must surely be a danger that one set of assumptions is merely replaced with another. Mezirow cites Habermas who has clearly recognised this fact:

> 'We are never in a position to know with absolute certainty that critical enlightenment has been effective, that it has liberated us from the ideological frozen constraints of the past, and initiated genuine self-reflection ... any claim of enlightened understanding may itself be a deeper and subtler form of self-deception ...' (Habermas 1974, cited by Mezirow 1981, p. 8)

Such ideas are challenging for an emerging profession such as nursing, which has based much of its practice on ritual and routine in the past (Bevis 1982), and is only now attempting to look with critical insight on its practice (Leino-Kilpi 1990; Darbyshire *et al.* 1990; Darbyshire 1991; McCaugherty 1991a, 1991b, 1992a, 1992b).

The notion of reflection needing to be much more than a retrospective process is also identified by Goodman (1984). He studied the reflections of trainee teachers and asserts that for reflection to be meaningful it has to have depth. He suggests reflective levels, based on Van Manen's (1977) work. Level one is concerned with the techniques needed to reach a given objective. At this level of reflection students are concerned with 'what works'. At level two they focus on the relationship between theory and practice. The third level incorporates reflections on both ethical and political concerns, and principles such as justice, equality and emancipation are used as criteria in deliberations (Goodman 1984). Goodman's concerns about the nature of teachers' reflections were also later shared by Calderhead who found that:

> 'student teachers' understanding and critical appraisal of their own and others' teaching was generally superficial and pragmatically orientated ... Reflection focused on the immediate concerns of accomplishing the task ahead of them.' (Calderhead 1989, p. 276)

These findings indicated that student teachers did not reflect in depth. Rather, they were concerned with getting on with day to day practice. While Goodman (1984) and Calderhead (1987) specifically examined the role of reflection in teacher education, my own research findings indicate that they are applicable to nursing also. While many expert nurses believed they were reflective, this was found to be at a superficial level only. Critical reflective abilities were the hallmark of the experts described as humanistic existentialists. It was also found that it was not the mechanical process of reflecting on practice that was crucial to enhancing practice; rather, it was the values, beliefs and knowledge bases which informed the reflective process that were significant. Also, reflection was found to be effective in transforming practice when expert nurses had the confidence to challenge themselves and others in a non-defensive but assertive manner (Conway 1996).

Providing a reflective culture

Through my work I have identified a number of factors which contribute to a culture that facilitates the development of reflective skills (Conway 1995). These include supportive environments where practitioners are encouraged to value themselves and their nursing skills. The establishment of relationships where practitioners could explore in safety the situations and events with which they had experienced difficulties also fostered the development of reflective skills.

The way work is organised is also influential. Primary nursing, for example, placed extra demands on nurses. These in turn required them to extend their knowledge bases. For reflection to be able to transform practice it needs to be put into action and often involves a challenging process. In some areas the skill of challenging effectively was actively encouraged. These areas of influence are clearly illustrated in the following exemplars.

Supporting others to transform nursing

An expert nurse described a situation which has several transformative aspects:

> I had a student working with me a few weeks ago – an undergraduate – and her lack of self worth was extraordinary. She could not see how she could contribute in any way whatsoever ... she had not had any general nursing experience, although ... in the third year of her degree ... and obviously she is very diffident about being on an acute medical ward ... you know lots of patients whizzing in and out ... and lines and drips, all the rest of it and ... helping some eat.
>
> This depressed lady, very depressed, did not want to eat at all, and ... needed someone to sit and cajole her and just be warm and talk and chatter and all the rest of it. I got her to focus on working with this person, sat with her for a little while, just to give her support and then just sort of went away for ten minutes and then came back and by the end of the day she had got this lady to smile.
>
> Now for her that was extraordinary you know ... getting somebody who was very, very depressed to smile, to eat, to drink and you know that was great because I was able to then ... [convey] the potential of the very ordinariness of nursing [to be] ... extraordinary in itself...
>
> Yes, you can go and slap a wet flannel all over someone and they will be washed, but you can also spend ten minutes ... Do it really really gently, make sure that you don't walk out of the room ... be really respectful of them, be really, really, gentle of them, make sure that what happens is what they want to happen, all those sorts of things and you have made a very very meaningful therapeutic interaction. Nursing at that level is extraordinary and is extraordinarily powerful.

The expert nurse supported and encouraged the student, helping her to transform her feelings about herself. In turn she was able to make a significant difference to the patient. Importance was attached to bringing caring and commitment to the nurse–patient interaction and it was this relationship that was transformative, not the task that the nurse carried out. It was not only students that were supported in this way. The expert nurse described the use of support networks amongst colleagues.

> We talk about ... things. About relationships, building relationships, and we do that with each other; that is not a hierarchical one-way street, we talk to each other about what we are doing.

This emphasis on open dialogue formed part of an ethos which fostered reflectivity. The notion of critical friendship further facilitated this process.

> I think it is important for all of us to have people, not necessarily the same person all the way through, and not necessarily one person to the exclusion of other people. We have got it to an extent already in devolving close relationships between colleagues ... so that you have got fewer close relationships ... we had a team meeting last night and [I] got home and said to my wife, I feel far less like a team leader nowadays, I feel like a team member, which is a really nice feeling to have. But the point is that at my ... organisational level, a G grade, I am giving to and gaining from four other people who are involved. So you are condensing the relationships; they are not as diluted as they would have been under the traditional model, whereas [as] a charge nurse I would have had to think about 20 odd people ... but we are sharing all that around and we are using ourselves to support people in doing that. (expert nurse)

While support and dialogue were seen as means of developing practitioners, there was also recognition that the care delivery method posed special challenges.

> You are encouraged in this environment to look at your effectiveness as a nurse and that includes your personal effectiveness as well as your external professional effectiveness ... that challenge has come from primary nursing ... it is the impetus from working closely with the client and the demands that relationship makes on the nurse ... she feels '[if] I am going to enter into this relationship, be this close, I need to know more than I currently do'. The exposure of educational need is very acute, is very sharply felt by the nurse when she is in that relationship with the patient. (Expert nurse, surgical area).

The experts described as humanistic existentialists (Conway 1995, 1996) integrated reflection into their working practices. Practitioners shared incidents in an effort to find strategies for the future. This often went beyond simple problem solving and required nurses to question their role and the role of others. This is illustrated in the following example where an expert nurse described an incident a colleague had discussed with him. The colleague was concerned that a patient was still for 222 (resuscitation) even though she was almost dead. The doctors involved were junior and did not want to make a decision. The expert explained that:

> The nurse on the other hand was thinking about it in terms of this person's quality of life ... [She was] trying to take their wishes into account, which was very difficult because the patient was virtually moribund anyway ... but [she] was then stuck in a dilemma of actually knowing that person was still for 222 ...
>
> [The patient] arrested in the middle of the night and she was stuck with this dilemma of knowing ... that it was an awful thing to have to do, but knowing that legally as far as she knew, [she] was bound to do it, which left her feeling very very sick indeed. (expert nurse)

Incidents such as this unfortunately are not uncommon in nursing. As detached observers it is easy to decide that a nurse should be more assertive in a given situation.

Encouraging assertiveness

This point was explored by the expert and the nurse involved.

> She ... [knew] the importance of being assertive ... but it isn't always so easy. I think probably the importance of actually sticking to a reasoned argument and also trying to make the opportunity for those debates to take place ... that was one of the things that ... instead of the nurses and the doctors who were looking after that patient getting together and talking it over as a group, you were getting a nurse coming on a shift being concerned about the situation, taking it up with one of the medical team who would then not feel empowered to make a decision because it was a difficult decision, who would then not make a decision because of the hundreds of other things, plus the socialisation of doctors which makes them conform, [and they] would not actually take that any further.
>
> So ... it was like a repeated situation rather than a situation that was growing. I think [what] ... came out strongly for her and for me was the fact that ... we ... [had to] to try to ... [develop] some process, you know sort of say [to the doctors] 'this is the policy guys for talking about resuscitation'. (expert nurse)

This discussion enabled the nurse to explore the issues in a non-threatening way. Also, importantly strategies for dealing with similar situations were developed. These strategies took account of the political nature of the relationship between doctors and nurses and sought, through asserting the nursing role in this process, to influence future practice. Reflection in this instance therefore facilitated personal and professional growth.

Developing challenging skills

Critical reflection on practice can often reveal that events and situations need challenging. This can be difficult for many nurses, particularly those who work in environments where they are not encouraged to ask questions but to get on with the work (Conway 1996). However, the ability to challenge yourself and others is integral to developing critical reflective skills. The humanistic existentialist experts (Conway 1996) actively encouraged others to develop challenging skills. A lecturer practitioner described her role in this process:

> I speak to the staff very regularly ... and that gives them a formal opportunity to raise concerns and quite often we plan out how a challenge might go: 'have you thought of presenting it this way?'. They tend to be terribly skilled and sensitive with patients, so when I say to them 'do you have the skills for challenging in a very sensitive and careful way so that people will listen to you? Look at the way that you broach bad news with patients, you are doing it in a very sensitive way. You could turn that to your colleagues'; and they suddenly think, 'yes I can do it' and that gives them a certain degree of confidence that they could tackle it and then we sort of talk over the worst scenario. You know, if you want to say this, what is the worst to the best and then they go [and] do it, and come and tell you about it and they will say, marvellous, marvellous, or whatever, and that way, if one or two instances are seen to be successful then it breeds an atmosphere where it is comfortable.

Practice such as this provides the opportunity for practitioners to gain skills in a supportive environment. They learn not only that it is acceptable to make challenges but indeed that challenges are expected of them. They are encouraged to look at how they are already providing care and to transfer some of these skills to the process of challenging. A challenge as presented in the scenario is not something practitioners have to steel themselves to do. Rather, it is about building their confidence in themselves, so that they can consider the worst possible consequences of an event and plan for it.

Transforming nursing through reflective attitudes

Another expert described an incident which illustrates clearly how nursing which is open, caring, and non judgemental can bring about change in even very difficult situations, making them manageable:

> A lot of things that stick in my mind are like transformative situations. I suppose some of my expertise is in recognising some situations as transformative and illuminating them ... For example, quite a few months ago we had a young man on the ward who had been in an RTA. He was wasted, contracted, he came to us from a rehabilitation unit because he was dehydrated and he had an infection and he became quite physically ill...
> Now the handover that we were given clearly labelled his partner as a trouble maker; we had comments like, 'don't let her interfere' and 'she will

take control, she will take over'. Which obviously said to me straight away, you want control, that's why you feel uncomfortable with her wanting control ... there were a couple of us that were intimately involved in the first few days.

What we did was, we just accepted her anxieties, so rather than trying to challenge her protectiveness, her anxieties, we tried very consciously, the two of us, to accept that that was a legitimate feeling under the circumstances ... she really wanted to be there for him and we converted a sense of being threatened by her wanting to have a degree of control and involvement in his care, to actually using that energy, transforming her emotion into something we would all be working with together ... and just recently we were invited to their wedding. We definitely made a significant difference, you could see her relax and start to trust, by listening to her ...

We were actually saying we agree with you, you have had a bit of a bad deal. We accept that you want to spend a lot of time with him, we accept that often you will know how to care for him best and certainly you understand and communicate better than we will ... of course we are experts in our field and we know about nutrition and we know about hydration and we know about the importance of these things; we know about gastrostomy tubes and we know about pressure sores but none of that is knowledge we can't teach to someone else.

There is no point in being jealous of that professional knowledge. I don't see any of us as being the sorts of people that would hold anything back. We don't want to use knowledge as power ... She was quite happy to trust him to our care and she actually had a rest which I thought was very good.

In such a situation it could be all too easy to label the patient's partner as a trouble maker. This would deny the real distress she was experiencing and ensure that, at best, care provision would be superficial only. The expert nurse's response, however, went far beyond this. It was at both an emotional and practical level. The expert nurse explained:

In that particular exemplar I am not just talking about sharing knowledge there was also an emotional response. Both of us that were involved in looking after that particular young man and woman in that early situation, were very aware of feeling her distress. We very much saw that as a focus for our care.

So our care, which my boss would actually see as something coming out of Buddhism, can also be seen as coming out of humanism, the idea of actually confronting anxiety, distress, negative fear and trying by one's own goodwill ... [to accept it] ... I was trying to respond in a human way to the suffering that was going on ... I know that I feel things very strongly in certain situations and I know that my colleagues do as well.

The transformative aspects of this situation are inextricably linked to the nurse's beliefs and values and how these are demonstrated in her attitude to the patient and his partner. Nursing in this situation is about conveying feelings. It is about responding in a caring human way to the situation.

Conclusion

It can be seen from the exemplars provided above that it is possible to assist practitioners to transform their practice. Fundamental to this is the development of a culture that fosters the development of critical thinking practitioners. The exemplars were all taken from nurses who work in environments where management positively support them. They all had authority to carry out their nursing actions. They were knowledgeable, indeed passionate about keeping a holistic nursing focus to practice. Educationally they were all well developed. Their beliefs and values were truly patient centred. The culture encouraged these nurses to reflect on their own practice. They were expected to have insight at a professional as well as a personal level. These nurses all carried their own case load of patients. They role modelled in practice what it meant to be critically reflective. They demonstrated very powerful nursing and showed through example how to transform nursing care. It is hoped that their experiences will inspire others to reflect on their practice and develop their own strategies for transforming it. It is also hoped that management will support such initiatives. If we really wish to provide high quality nursing care, providing a culture where such care flourishes is one way this can be accomplished.

References

Bevis, E.O. (1982) Conceptual framework: philosophical base. *Curriculum Building in Nursing a Process*, 3rd edn, pp. 35–55. St. Louis, Mosby.

Boud, D., Keogh, R. & Walker D. (eds.) (1985) *Reflection: Turning Experience into Learning*. Kogan Page, London.

Calderhead, J. (1989) Reflective teaching and teacher education. *Teaching and Teacher Education*, 5, 43–51.

Carr, W. & Kemmis, S. (1986) *Becoming Critical: Education Knowledge and Action Research*. Falmer Press, London.

Conway, J.E. (1995) *Expert nursing knowledge as an evolutionary process*. Unpublished PhD thesis. University of Warwick, Coventry.

Conway, J.E. (1996) *Nursing Expertise and Advanced Practice*. Quay Books Division, Mark Allen Publishers, Salisbury.

Darbyshire, P., Stewart, B., Jamieson, I. & Tongue, C. (1990) New domains in nursing. *Nursing Times*, **86**(27), 73–5.

Darbyshire, P. (1991) Nursing reflections. *Nursing Times*, **87**(36), 27–8.

Dewey, J. (1933) *How we Think: a Restatement of the Relation of Reflective Thinking to the Educational Process*. D.C. Heath and Co, London.

FEU (1981) *Experience, Reflection, Learning*. Department of Education and Science, Further Education Curriculum and Development Unit, London.

Freire, P. (1970) *Cultural Action for Freedom*. Penguin Books, Harmondsworth.

Goodman, J. (1984) Reflection and teacher education: a case study and theoretical analysis. *Interchange*, 15, 9–25.

Habermas, J. (1974) *Theory and Practice*. Heinemann, London.

Leino-Kilpi, H. (1990) Self-reflection in nursing teacher education. *Journal of Advanced Nursing*, 15, 192–5.

McCaugherty, D. (1991a) The theory–practice gap in nurse education: its causes and possible solutions. Findings from an action research study. *Journal of Advanced Nursing*, 16, 1055–61.

McCaugherty, D. (1991b) The use of a teaching model to promote reflection and the experiential integration of theory and practice in first year student nurses: an action research study. *Journal of Advanced Nursing*, May, 165, 534–43.

McCaugherty, D. (1992a) The gap between nursing theory and practice. *Senior Nurse*, 12(6), 44–8.

McCaugherty, D. (1992b) The concepts of theory and practice. *Senior Nurse*, 30(122), 29–33.

Mezirow, J. (1981) A critical theory of adult learning and education. *Adult Education*, 32(1), 3–24.

Schön, D.A. (1983) *The Reflective Practitioner: How Professionals Think in Action.* Basic Books Inc., New York.

Schön, D.A. (1987) *Educating the Reflective Practitioner.* Jossey-Bass, London.

Van Manen, M. (1977) Linking ways of knowing with ways of being practical. *Curriculum Inquiry*, 6(3), 205–28.

Chapter 13

Reflective Practice – a Way to the Patient's World and Caring, the Core of Nursing

Tina Nordman, Anne Kasén and Katie Eriksson

Introduction

In this chapter we have used an ontological caring–scientific ideal model as a starting-point for reflective practice in order to capture the pattern of the patient's conception of the caring reality. Reflective practice in caring nursing presupposes a special kind of perspective. The perspective decides the direction of the reflection and its substance is based on a caring science perspective; it is based both on an ontological and a scientific ideal. A reflection which has no clear perspective may become technical and empty and it may even miss its actual purpose.

Nursing care may be transformed into caring through reflective practice. Nursing care without caring becomes empty and meaningless unless we are able to reflect upon the evident things in care. To reflect is to ponder over the visible reality and to break through the surface in order to reach deeper spheres where the idea of caring can be found. The reflection is based on the patient's conception of reality. The patient is a person who suffers and endures something. A human being who suffers also changes and suffering may either lead to death or a new life (Eriksson 1993; Lindholm & Eriksson 1993). Surprisingly little research has been carried out in caring from the point of view of the patient. It therefore felt important to research caring which reflected the patient's conception of reality.

Nursing research has been criticised for not discussing or taking into consideration the connection between ontology, methodology and epistemology (Eriksson 1994; Koch 1995). The ontology of caring science indicates the general outlines of possible methodology (Boykin & Schoenhofer 1993; Eriksson 1996).

An autonomous caring science develops its ontology and epistemology in interaction with practice. The ideal model of caring science is based on its ontology and it involves a dynamic perspective. The model is continuously developing in relation to ongoing scientific research. The ideal model (Eriksson 1987a, b) has developed during a time when the autonomous caring science developed and tried to find its place in the scientific world. The research which the ideal model is based on has mainly been basic research which develops concepts and substance related to caring. Today, the main focus is clinical caring science research which has its starting-point in caring science as a field of science (Eriksson 1996).

When we choose caring science as a field of science, we regard caring science as an autonomous science. To have an ideal model is to look at reality from a special point of view (Alvesson & Skjûldberg 1994). The ideal model represents a special form of abductive hypothesis, i.e. the idea of what reality could be like, which helps us find the meaningful deep structures in the the field of research. If we choose a field of research as our starting-point, we do not have an explicit model controlling our research. This means that the research results may remain at a superficial level and be of advantage to other sciences than caring science.

In order to get a description of the patient's conception of reality as a basis for authentic care, we brought out an example from caring science research where reflective practice is based on the ontology of caring science.

The Department of Caring Science at Åbo Akademy University in Finland has initiated clinical research in caring by the research programme 'In the patient's world, a study of health, suffering and caring'. The emphasis in the different projects of the research programme is based on the ideal model and earlier research (Eriksson 1993; Eriksson *et al.* 1995; Kasén 1994; Lindström 1995; Nordman 1995).

Some basic beliefs have been formulated:

(1)   The human being is a whole of body, soul and spirit
(2)   The human suffering is a starting-point for caring
(3)   Health is more than absence of illness. To be healthy is to be whole, to experience and feel whole as regards body, soul, and spirit. Health is part of life. Health has no meaning unless life has meaning. Health is consistent with endurable suffering.
(4)   Caring is based on the motive of caritas (see Chapter 18), which through compassion awakens a desire to alleviate another's suffering.

We have to be aware of the caring–scientific ontology which is used, otherwise it may become an obstacle in our research. It should rather be its starting-point and a connecting thought throughout research and reflection.

Caring – the core of nursing

Caring is based on the motive of caritas, which has its historical origin in the ideals of mercy and maternity. The preliminary substance of caring is faith, hope and love, which are fundamental sources of strength for human beings. This substance is developed through caring by purging, playing and learning. Purging is the most primary form aiming at pleasure; playing aims at trust, and learning aims at development. The significance of the context of caring is caring communion (Eriksson 1994). The caring relationship is the basic motive of caring. The patient is invited and received in a caring relationship and his/her dignity is confirmed. The nurse talks to, touches, the suffering human being in the relationship (Eriksson 1995, p. 27). The substance of the caring relationship is the patient's story, which is created when the nurse becomes part of it (Kasén 1994).

Different forms of suffering have been indicated in caring (Eriksson 1993; Lindholm & Eriksson 1993). These are suffering related to illness, suffering related to care, and suffering related to life. Suffering related to illness has to do with experiences related to illness and treatment. Suffering related to care is about experiences related to nursing situations. Suffering related to life is about experiences in individual life. When suffering gets the better of a person, he/she gradually 'disappears' – first his/her mental and spiritual dimensions and, finally, his/her body. When suffering leads to a new life, man has reconciled himself to his life and suffering has been given meaning, because suffering itself has no meaning. The patient can encounter the nurse in the caring communion as a co-actor in the drama of suffering. The nurse is keenly aware of the patient's experiences of suffering, which may be expressed in the forms of symbols and metaphors. When the nurse suffers together with the patient the patient can conceive suffering as meaningful.

Suffering aims at health, which consists with endurable suffering. Health and suffering converge deep down in man's inner entity, which is expressed by his body, soul and spirit. Health is becoming, which is the core of the ontological health model (Eriksson *et al.* 1995; Herberts & Eriksson 1995). Caring reaches beyond health; it makes a human being become the person he was intended to be.

Three nursing traditions which express different patterns of caring reality

The caring reality is complex. In the course of history, caring has been affected by the development of society as well as by the development of different sciences, especially medicine. Caring takes place in an ethical and cultural context. It is about encounters between patients and nurses in different situations of caring reality, where the extent of the nurse's ethical responsibility emerges. When man's dignity as a manifestation of his uniqueness is confirmed, a basic category in the ethics of caring has been fulfilled (Eriksson 1995, p. 25). Different caring cultures can be discovered in the caring reality in the form of nursing traditions (Eriksson 1996). These traditions provide a basis when we want to reflect upon the idea of caring and they also elucidate the perspective of caring science in the caring reality as well as in research.

The different nursing traditions have different resources of concepts and are based on different research traditions (Fig. 13.1). The concepts we use reflect the researcher's conception of the world and of science. An autonomous caring science presupposes concepts which are consistent with the ontology of caring science (Eriksson 1996).

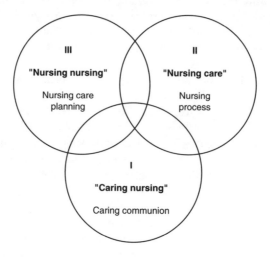

Fig. 13.1   Caring and nursing perspectives.

Nursing I (caring nursing) describes the innermost part of caring. This is a kind of caring which without prejudice aims to put the patient and his/her suffering and needs in the first place. This care may seem unstructrured and chaotic from the outside, but its inner structure reponds to good and individual patient care. The caring relation is a form of communion and the caring profile is caritas (Eriksson 1992). Nursing II (nursing care) is based on the nursing process and it aims to systematically respond to the patient's needs. The reasoning is here based on illness and diagnosis. This kind of nursing becomes good care when it is controlled by the innermost part of caring. However, if the innermost part is not taken into consideration, nursing may be techni-cally good but it is not caring. Nursing III (nursing nursing) is based on the structures of nursing care planning and its aim is a systematic planning of patient care. Unless it is based on the nursing process and the essence of nursing, there is a risk that nursing becomes an admin-istrative structure without caring substance. Good nursing, which aims at total care, must include all three perspectives mentioned (Eriksson 1996).

These three 'nursing' traditions imply that there are three different worlds and cultures in the clinical nursing reality. It also means that there are three different traditions of science and research. Each tradition is based on different ontologies and conceptual models. We need methods which can penetrate into different levels of reality so that we can discover different nursing traditions. Reflective interpretation is such a method.

Reflective interpretation

The method in the project 'In the patient's world' has been reflective interpretation (Alvesson & Skjöldberg 1994) with an abductive and hermeneutical design (Gadamer 1988). The abductive approach makes it possible to seek possibilities and to broaden the evident, whereas hermeneutics is represented by a deepening spiral.

Empirical research is characterised by reflection on the evident and it tries to find understanding, not to establish truths (Alvesson & Skjöldberg 1994, p. 12). The chosen method implies that the researcher is open-minded and that he/she uses the method flexibly in relation to the purpose of the study. The method cannot define in advance what we should seek; it only indicates the general outlines for the search (Alvesson & Skjöldberg 1994; Gadamer 1988).

The different elements of the reflection are the movement, width and variation. Movement means that it is possible to move on different levels of knowledge in the reflection from an ontological to an empirical level. It is also a movement between the different aspects of reflective interpretation. These are made up of the nearness to the empirical material, hermeneutics, a critical approach and self-criticism, or a further seeking for levels based on the material found.

The hermeneutical spiral is a symbol for continuously deepening movement. The width of the reflection is the interpreter's ability to use different repertoires of interpretation. A broad body of knowledge makes variation possible in the reflection. (Alvesson & Skjöldberg 1994, pp. 324–5).

Interpretation means that you have a dialogue with the text, probe it, and ask it questions so that it talks to you. The interpreter seeks the underlying question/metaphor, to which the text provides a key. Common sense helps you to discover the right question. The interpreter keeps at a certain distance from his prejudices and can in the process move deeper down the hermeneutical spiral. The question indicates the horizon where the meaning of the text can be captured. (Alvesson & Skjöldberg 1994; Gadamer 1988).

The abductive approach means that a separate case is interpreted in relation to a hypothetical or possible pattern, which may be an ideal image. The caring–scientific ideal image is here the pattern of abductive interpretation. The overall horizon of the abductive approach is understanding (Alvesson & Skjöldberg 1994, p. 42). The interpreter 'takes a leap' over the evident through the empirical material and theories. Silva *et al.* (1995) talk about knowledge on-beyond which lies beyond the tangible, and such knowledge can be reached through an abductive approach.

Our reflection has its starting-point in the caring–scientific ideal image, which serves as a tool between ontology and empiricism. The material which the interpretation is based on has been gathered by means of diaries, unstructured observation and discussions with patients (Eriksson 1993; Eriksson *et al.* 1995; Kasén 1994; Lindström 1995; Nordman 1995). The validity is guaranteed through researchers' triangulation and triangulation in method when gathering the data. The selection is based on material from the project 'In the patient's world' from which we have chosen different patients in order to be able to illustrate reflective interpretation.

Reflective interpretation adapted to the material is illustrated in Fig. 13.2. We begin with the empirical material and ask the text what the

---

A picture of the interpretation perspectives and the interpretation process

The patient expresses that he is satisfied, but also nervous, concerning the stay in hospital. The patient feels there is tension, also that there is promise and the hope of getting well in the hospital. The days in the hospital go by but the promise is not fulfilled. The patient is just as full of expectation every day, but he becomes disappointed again, because this day he did not meet anybody who could have helped him. The food is good and a great many examinations are being made, which the patient thinks is good. However, the patient thinks that many things could be improved in the care. He makes suggestions but they are not heeded.

Experience
Nervous – tension – promise – possibility – expectation – disappointment – satisfaction (food) – hope – nobody listens

Metaphor
I had no playing time

Level III
The patient is satisfied with the care

Level II
The patient adjusts himself to his nursing programme, to examinations which presuppose that the patient has a diagnosed illness. The patient does not have a diagnosed illness which makes it difficult to find him the right nursing programme. The patient is a hopeless case. The measurable dimensions of health are in the forefront. Health is a doing.

Level I
The patient experiences suffering related to care when he is not invited to the caring communion as an entity of body, soul and spirit. The patient has been reduced to a diagnosis instead of being encountered as a patient who suffers. His will and wish to be part of the care are strong, but the patient feels that he is disregarded when nobody listens to him. In spite of this, the patient still feels hope. The underlying metaphor is 'I had no playing time'. The patient is somebody who endures and suffers something (Eriksson 1993, 1994). Balance and harmony are elements in health as a being (Eriksson 1993, p. 15). Since hope is one of man's basic qualities, the patient can endure the suffering related to care and this makes it possible to experience unmeasurable health.

Fig. 13.2   The patient's conceptions of reality.

patient experiences. We now have a dialogue with the text and try to find the underlying metaphor of every text. The different interpretation perspectives make up the different stages of our interpretation. Interpretation perspective III exemplifies the most superficial level, interpretation perspective II exemplifies the following stage of the interpretation when we have penetrated below the surface, whereas interpretation perspective I is the deepest level where the unerlying metaphor is found. The different interpretation perspectives can be compared with the different nursing traditions. The underlying metaphor is then interpreted abductively in relation to the caring–scientific ideal image of suffering and health (Nygren 1972).

Pictures from the patient's reality

Reflective interpretation is illustrated below in order for us to understand the patient's reality in a deeper sense. The four examples capture patients' experiences of care based on different perspectives. In order to reach the unique experiences and by that means an idiographic pattern, we have used metaphors which have been captured in the interpretation process and which respond to the patient's reality.

I had no playing time

This patient expresses that he is satisfied, but also nervous concerning the care/the stay in hospital. The patient feels there is tension, also that there is promise and the hope of getting well in the hospital. The days in the hospital go by but the promise is not fulfilled. The patient is just as full of expectation every day, but he becomes disappointed again, because this day he did not meet anybody who could have helped him. The food is good and a great many examinations are being made, which the patient thinks is good. However, the patient thinks that many things could be improved in the care. He makes suggestions but they are not heeded.

On first reflection from interpretation of the example, we may understand that the patient has been satisfied after all (interpretation perspective III). When we approach the text again, we meet a patient who has been nervous about different examinations and who has been rather active regarding his own care. The patient is considered as a hopeless case since his diagnosis is still unclear in spite of the fact that different examinations have been made. The measurable dimensions of health are in the forefront (interpretation perspective II).

However, we are not satisfied with this interpretation, we continue our interpretation from a caring perspective (interpretation perspective I). The patient is not invited to the caring relationship as an entity of body, soul and spirit, and this gives rise to suffering related to care. The patient's will and wish to be included in the care are strong but the patient feels that he is not taken notice of as nobody listens to him. In spite of this, the patient still feels hope. The underlying methaphor is 'I had no playing time'. The patient is somebody who endures and suffers something (Eriksson 1993, & 1994). Balance and harmony are elements in health as a being (Eriksson 1993, p. 15). Since hope is one of man's basic qualities, the patient can endure the suffering related to care and this makes it possible to experience unmeasurable health.

I was deprived of my freedom

The patient says that he is satisfied with the care even though he was nervous when he arrived at the hospital. He thought that he would rest at the hospital since he could not work there. He drew the curtains round his bed in the patient's room and did not want to be disturbed. Despite this he felt his fellow patients did not leave him alone. The nurses are kind and nice when they come to the patient to perform some duty, but they are continuosly coming and going and this disturbs the patient. The noise from the corridor penetrates through the wall and the patient says that it gives him a headache. The people around the patient do not leave him in peace. The experiences of the 'room' become more and more stressing, even suffocating. The patient says that he must go home in order to rest.

The text interpreted on a superficial level (interpreted perspective III) tells us that the patient has been fairly satisfied with the care that he has received. When we continue to interpret it, we ask the text what the patient has experienced. The answer is that the patient is calm and reserved; the only thing he complained of was headache (health as the opposite of illness), for which he was prescribed medicine (interpretation perspective II).

Interpretation perspective I gives us the message that this patient has not had the right to be a patient in the original sense of the word, to suffer, since he is being disturbed all the time. None of the nurses respond to the patient's suffering, since the emphasis in the care is on the nursing activities that are to be carried out. The patient feels that the mental and spiritual space is too restricted, which means that he is unable to rest, to find a peace or breathing-space. The encroachment on the patient's integrity is an experience of being 'deprived of freedom', and this gives rise to a suffering related to care. To reduce health to headache is to emphaize health from external objective criteria, to see health as a doing (Herberts & Eriksson 1995). To have a place where you can rest alleviates suffering. To flee from suffering is a form of evil suffering (Eriksson 1993, p. 22). To provide the patient with some breathing-space means that he can find a meaning in suffering. When suffering is not strange to the patient, he can experience health as a doing.

I am an invisible child

This patient talks about the nursing routines. They are familiar to him and easy to identify. The patient feels that it is easier for him to adjust himself to the hospital when he knows these routines and follows them. They make him feel secure, but they also tie him down to the system of the ward at the hospital. The patient feels that nothing happens in between the different nursing measures; he just lies and waits. He is seized with longing and this makes him incapable of acting. He feels that he has to adjust to the system but he still wonders whether it serves its purpose or not. This patient does not have the courage to call the care into question; he 'lies quietly' in his bed and waits. The patient has given up, other people are left to decide.

Again, we meet a satisfied patient in the text according to interpretation perspective III. It is profitable to nurse the patient since he has an illness for which there is a nursing programme (intrepretation perspective II).

The experiences that we find in the following interpretation are that the patient feels violated since he has been degraded and considered unworthy. He is a thing which waits for certain measures to be carried out. Caring then gives rise to a suffering related to care, violating the dignity of the unique human being. The patient does not want to 'disturb' the nurse; instead he gives up and leaves the responsibility for his health to a system. Deep down (interpretation perspective I) in the text we find the metaphor 'the invisible child'. To give up in suffering is a way of alleviating suffering. This is, however, evil suffering (Eriksson 1993, p. 22). The patient longs for the nurse to confirm him as he is, as an entity of body, soul and spirit. Suffering is lust (Eriksson 1993, p. 25). If we bear in mind the patient's longing as an expression of lust, we make it possible for the patient to ascribe some meaning to his suffering and thereby experience health.

You show me the way

In the following example we meet a patient who says that he has experienced the arrival in the ward as a sort of home-coming. He was received with respect for his uniqueness and he felt invited since the nurses welcomed him by taking his hand and looking happy. The patient immediately became familiar with the other patient in the room. The stay at the hospital was long and it also included a great many problems, such as pain and insomnia, but it was, however, safer to be at hospital than at home.

The patient says that he is satisfied with the care that he has received (interpretation perspective III). When the interpretation advances (perspective II), we meet a patient who has different illnesses and problems. The patient experiences that he has received adequate care for them.

In the following interpretation we find experiences of trust in the ward and in the hospital as well as experiences of being approved by nurses as well as by fellow patients as a separate unique individual. In spite of different difficult problems which gave rise to experiences of suffering related to illness and care, the patient experiences that the care is good. The metaphor (interpretation perspective I) is 'You show me the way'. To be confirmed is to meet a co-actor in the drama of suffering. The patient can by that means ascribe a meaning to suffering (Eriksson 1993, p. 14). Health as a becoming means that suffering is not strange to man (Eriksson 1993, p. 15). Through the drama of suffering the patient can experience that the suffering is a natural part of man's health.

The drama of suffering as the patient's reality

It is difficult to verbalise suffering and therefore it is expressed in other ways, as metaphors (Lindholm & Eriksson 1993; Younger 1995). This is why it is central to take into consideration the patient's different ways of expressing himself. To confirm suffering is the first stage in the drama of suffering.

The second act in the drama of suffering is to give the patient the time and the space he needs to suffer (Lindholm & Eriksson 1993). This means that the patient is not left alone, he has a co-actor in the drama; otherwise, he will experience suffering related to care as in 'the invisible child'. To experience the meaning of suffering means that you have possibilities (Eriksson 1993, p. 18). What kind of possibilities can a patient be offered by care? The nurse should discover these possibilities together with the patient, otherwise his reality will be suffocated in such a way as the patient in the text 'No playing time'. The patient creates the space together with the nurse in the caring communion, which also reflects the two other nursing traditions (II and III). The patient can freely express his wishes and the promise of help can be fulfilled in a meaningful caring relationship. The patient can ascribe some meaning to his suffering in this relationship, since the nurse suffers with him. This is how the patient can keep his hope, faith and love as fundamental sources of strength in order to be able to advance towards a higher degree of integrated health. A caring culture which reflects the true nature of caring gives the nurse the freedom to act for the patient's own good. Her actions aim to serve the other, the patient, and to encounter him with dignity which gives him strength to shape his own life (Eriksson 1994).

The third act in the drama of suffering is reconciliation and a way to a new entity. The patient's dignity as a human being is confirmed when the nurse shows him respect. This is how the patient is provided with the breathing-space which makes it possible for him to use his own vitality and his courage to face life. He can then develop the mission which belongs to the human being. Suffering is consistent with health (Eriksson 1993, p. 15). When caring is merely technical without caring substance, the patient gets support for the measurable dimensions of health. To reduce the patient's health to illness is to totally neglect the patient's resources and to forget the overall view of health (Lindsey 1996). To regard health as a whole is to take all human dimensions, body, soul and spirit, into consideration. The experience of health on a level of becoming is an experience of the spiritual dimension of the human entity (Herberts & Eriksson 1995; Lindsey 1996).

The results of our interpretation show that there is a dialectic in the patients' experiences, they all include experiences of the good as well as the bad care. Bad care includes experiences of, for instance, suffering related to care, and good care includes experiences of caritative care. The patients' experiences (parts) must be related to the whole of the individual unique patient in order for us to be able to decide where the main focus of the experiences is, on the good or on the bad.

In addition to the dialectic, the patient's wishes also emerged. The nurse gains knowledge about the patient's wishes by reflecting upon the things which seems 'self-evident'. In this reflection, the patient appears the way he is as a suffering human being. By responding to the patient's wishes, it is possible for the nurse to join the drama of suffering together with the patient. The wishes are a way to deeper understanding of the patient's experiences of care. A nursing tradition which cultivates the idea of caring can respond to the patient's demands/desires in a better way.

What do the patient's wishes reflect? They reflect that there should be a concrete other person who can confirm the patient in the caring communion. The patient can reconcile himself to suffering related to care if his dignity as a human being is confirmed.

Where has our reflection brought us?

We have sought a pattern for good care. Our starting-points have been the patient's conception of reality and the idea of caring on an ontological level. We have used reflective practice on meaningful material, which is made up of the patient's experiences of care from the project 'In the patient's world'.

We emphasise that the primary quality of good care can only be captured by asking the patients. Reflective interpretation is a method which can be used to capture the pattern for good care. The ontology of caring science determines the method as well as the frame of the interpretation. We emphasise that it is a matter of decisive importance that caring–scientific research should be based on its own ontology, because otherwise we cannot develop a pattern for good care from our own perspective.

A given caring culture may stagnate unless we are eager to change it. The culture should also provide the nurse with freedom and security so that she can reflect (Palmer 1994; Rodgers 1994). The nurse's perspective is shaped by habits and traditions and her perspective will stagnate unless there is reflection. A random act must become conscious in order for continuous and directed development of the substance of caring to take place. (Eriksson 1996).

A caritative culture is synthesis of all the different nursing traditions. In such culture, it is possible for the nurse to cultivate cultural goods which emphasise the idea of caring. The human being as an entity of body, soul and spirit is a patient in the original sense of the word, i.e. somebody who endures and suffers something. This person's entity encounters the nurse's entity as a co-actor in the drama of suffering. The patient can ascribe some meaning to suffering in spite of different experiences of suffering related to care. This is how he or she begins/continues the process towards a new integrated entity of health as a becoming, where suffering and health are a natural part of life. The patient's unbearable suffering can only be alleviated in a caring communion where the nurse confirms his/her suffering. The nurse invites the patient to the caring communion where caring without demands creates space for the patient where he/she can rest and find peace. This allows the patient's own vitality to grow (Eriksson 1994, 1995).

The complex caring reality consists of different nursing traditions which in different ways express the idea of caring. The idea of caring which extends through the different levels and structures supports the development of the caring reality. This is how the patient's concept of reality becomes the starting-point for development.

The nurse's motive to care is found in the caring motive (Eriksson 1992). The nurse gets the strength to be a co-actor in the process. When the caring culture prevails, not only in a specific ward but throughout a whole organisation, the nurse is able to grow and develop. When the nurse is aware of her caring–scientific paradigm, she can use it as a means of assistance in reflective interpretation, since her reflection can take place in a wider sense. This means that the nurse can discover meaningful questions based on the ontology of caring science in the caring reality. In the clinical caring reality, we have to discover questions about the patient's conception of reality, and through reflective inter-pretation reach a higher degree of understanding of the patient. Care, nursing care, may become a technical job in which the nurse only carries out tasks. This job will lack the idea of caring unless the nurse makes use of the creative pause in care. The substance of care arises when a caring situation is created. It is characterised by the interaction between reflection and production (Eriksson 1987a, p. 15). Caring becomes a skill instead of a technical action when man's dignity and entity are con-firmed (Eriksson 1996).

In order to support the development of the caring reality we need caring science research focusing on the patient's perspective (Munhall 1995; Thomas & Bond 1996). Research on the patient's perspective is changing from a nomothetic perspective to an idiographic one where the experiences of the unique patient are sought. It is important to change the perspective and bring out the actual experiences of the patients in order to develop care (Thomas & Bond 1996; Price 1996). If we are going to develop an overall pattern for good nursing care, we also need the patient's perspective.

Several authors call attention to the connection between the ontology of caring science, epistemology, and methodology (Silva *et al.* 1995; Walters 1995). The literature emphasises the importance of analysing central concepts in care. It is a matter of decisive importance that the development is determined by the representatives of caring science (Wurzbach 1996). The concepts which are used must be consistent with the hard-core of caring science. Bishop & Scudder (1995) consider that nursing is reduced to concerning only the nursing of the sick in case nursing is compared to interventions. Caring is the core of nursing and it is characterised by a being, not by carrying out tasks (Nelms 1996). We need research which is based on a wider view of health, where health is regraded as something more than the opposite of illness (Thompson *et al.* 1995). The ontological health model of caring science (Eriksson *et al.* 1995; Herberts & Eriksson 1995) reflects an overall view on health.

We also have to try out different methods, especially methods which emphasise deep structures. Reflective practice in care is also of immediate importance. However, we call attention to the fact that the reflection must be based on the ontology of caring science, so that we can penetrate into caring reality. Clarke *et al.* (1996) call attention to technical/practical, personal and structural aspects. We realise that we have to penetrate even deeper into the caring reality and discover the idea of caring. Silva *et al.* (1995) talk about knowledge on-beyond. The complexity of the caring reality requires reflection upon the visible towards the possible. The abductive conclusion captures the possible.

When the nurse's reflection is based on the idea of caring, the perspective becomes understanding and humanistic. Its central methods are the circle or the dialogue (Boykin & Schoenhofer 1993). Hermeneutical reflection is a method for all of us in the caring reality (Walters 1995).

The criteria of validity and reliability vary depending on which tradition research is based on. Caring science belongs to the humanities, which means that the concept of truth indicates understanding (Eriksson 1991; Walters 1995). Relating the concept of truth to understanding means that we dissociate ourselves from exact truth. The result of hermeneutical research should provide us with knowledge which increases our underbtanding of reality. We must have the courage to try out methods and to interpret in order to capture knowledge which is meaningful for the development of caring science. Reflective interpretation has proved to be useful when we want to penetrate through superficial structures and reach underlying currents. The conclusions that have been drawn guide us in the following stage of the project and they are tried out through deduction and induction by means of methodic triangulation. The aim of the project is then to develop a kind of instrument out of the knowledge we obtained through our qualitative studies. The measuring intrument would function as a means and basis for evaluation in clinical practice. The results of the projects have also been used in education and further education, in seminars for students and nurses.

Another important criterion in reflective and explorative research is the wealth of aspects in relation to empiricism (Alvesson & Skjûldberg 1994, p. 358). Empirisicm serves as a starting-point and it should be possible to relate the interpretations and the conclusions obtained from the process to the basic material obtained from empiricism. We see that the metaphors exemplify the wealth of aspects. The metaphors speak a language which is not related to the verbal language.

Conclusion

The central theme of the reflective interpretation is movement. The interpretation has been verified by using different sources of material within the project 'In the patient's world'. The use of the different interpretation perspectives and suffering and health is a movement which in itself confirms the research results of the process. The movement and the self-criticism reduce the risk of the subjectivism. A hermeneutical interpretation should lead to a deepening spiral, not to a vicious circle (Helenius 1994; Ödman 1991).

The material and the method that we have used here are examples of the possibilities with which we can change the caring reality, but we do not only need tools, we also need visions. When we have visions in the caring reality, we also have the opportunity to develop it so that it responds to the patient's wishes in a better way. Otherwise, the caring reality will wither. Let us create possibilities of developing visions together.

References

Alvesson, M. & Skjöldberg, K. (1994) *Tolkning och reflektion*. Studentlitteraturen, Lund.

Bichop, A. & Scudder, J. (1995) Applied science, practice, and intervention technology. In *Search for Nursing Science* (eds A. Omrey, C. Kasper, G. Page), pp. 263–74. Sage Publication, London.

Boykin, A & Schoenhofer, S. (1993) *Nursing as Caring. A Model for Transforming Practice*. National League for Nursing Press, New York.

Clarke, B., James, C. & Kelly, J. (1996) Reflective practice: reviewing the issues and refocusing the debate. *International Journal of Nursing Studies*, 2,171–80.

Eriksson, K. (1987a) *Pausen*. Almqvist & Wiksell, Stockholm.

Eriksson, K. (1987b) *Vardandets ide*. Almqvist & Wiksell, Stockholm.

Eriksson, K. (1991) *Broar. Introduktion i vardvetenskaplig metod*. Department of Caring Science, Åbo Akademi, Vasa.

Eriksson, K. (1992) Nursing: The caring practice 'being there'. In *The Presence of Caring Nursing* (ed. D. Gaut), pp. 200–10. National League for Nursing Press, New York.

Eriksson, K. (1993) *Möten med lidanden.* Vardforskning 4/1993. Department of Caring Science, Åbo Akademi, Vasa.

Eriksson K. (1994) Theories of caring as health. In *Caring as Healing: Renewal through Hope* (ed. D. Gaut, & A. Boykin). National League for Nursing Press, New York.

Eriksson, K. (ed) (1995) *Mot en vardetik.* Vardforskning 5/1995. Department of Caring Science, Åbo Akademi, Vasa.

Eriksson, K. (ed), Bondas-Salonen, T., Herberts, S., Lindholm, L. & Matilainen, D. (1995) *Den mangdimensionella halsan– verklighet och visioner.* Slutrapport. Vasa sjukvardsdistrikt SKN och Institutionen för vardvetenskap, Åbo Akademi, Vasa.

Eriksson, K. (1996) Understanding the world of the patient, the suffering human being – the new clinical paradigm from nursing caring. Manuscript (accepted). *Advanced Practice Nursing Quarterly.*

Gadamer, H-G. (1988) *Truth and Method.* Sheed and Ward, London.

Helenius, R. (1994) *Första och bättre veta.* Carlssons, Stockholm.

Herberts, S. & Eriksson, K. (1995) Nursing leaders' and nurses' view of health. *Journal of Advanced Nursing,* 22, 868–78.

Kasén, A. (1994) *Vardrelationen-en begreppsanalytisk studie.* Master's thesis. Department of Caring Science, Åbo Akademi, Vasa.

Koch, T. (1995) Interpretive approaches in nursing research: the influence of Husserl and Heidegger. *Journal of Advanced Nursing,* 5, 827–36.

Lindholm, L. & Eriksson, K. (1993) To understand and alleviate sufffering in caring culture. *Journal of Advanced Nursing,* 18, 1354–61.

Lindsey, E. (1996) Health within illness: experiences of chrinically ill/disabled people. *Journal of Advanced Nursing,* 24, 465–72.

Lindström, U. (1995) Ensamhetskönslan sviker inte. Vardforskning/1995. Department of Caring Science, Åbo Akademi, Vasa.

Munhall, A. (1995) Nursing research: what difference does it make? *Journal of Advanced Nursing,* 21, 576–83.

Nelms, T. (1996) Living a caring presence in nursing: a Heideggerian hermeneutical analysis. *Journal of Advanced Nursing,* 24, 368–74.

Nordman, T. (1995) *Star tiden stilla? En empirisk undersökning av patienters upplevelser av caritativ vard pa sjukhus.* Master's thesis. Department of Caring Science, Åbo Akademi, Vasa.

Nygren, A. (1972) *Meaning and Method. Prolegomena to a Scientific Philosophy of Religion and a Scientific Theology.* Epworth Press, London.

Ödman, P-J. (1991) *Tolkning, förstaelse vetande. Hermeneutik i teori och prektik.* Almqvist & Wiksell, Stockholm.

Palmer, A. (1994) Introduction. In *Reflective Practice in Nursing: the Growth of the Professional Practitioner* (ed. A. Palmer, S. Burns & C. Bulman), pp. 1–9. Blackwell Science, Oxford.

Price, B. (1996) Illness careers: the chronic illness experience. *Journal of Advanced Nursing,* 24, 275–9.

Rodgers, S. (1994) An exploratory study of research utilization by nurses in general medical and surgical wards. *Journal of Advanced Nursing,* 20, 904–11.

Silva, M. & Merkle, J. & Sorrell, C. (1995) From Carper's pattern of knowing to ways of being: an ontological philosophical shift in nursing. *Advances in Nursing Science,* 1, 1–13.

Thomas, L. & Bond, S. (1996) Measuring patient's satisfaction with nursing: 1990–1994. *Journal of Advanced Nursing,* 23, 747–56.

Thompson, D., Steven, J. & Webster, R. (1995) The experiences of patients and their partners one month after a heart attack. *Journal of Advanced Nursing*, 22, 707–14.

Walters, A. (1995) The phenomenological movement: implications for nursing research. *Journal of Advanced Nursing*, 22, 791–9.

Wurzbach, M. (1996) Comfort and nurses' moral choices. *Journal of Advanced Nursing*, 24, 260–4.

Younger, J. (1995) The alienation of the sufferer. *Journal of Advanced Nursing*, 17, 53–72.

Chapter 14
The Philosopher's Stone

Dawn Freshwater

Introduction

Transformation literally means a change of shape, change of character – a metamorphosis; rather like the caterpillar, which after spending time incubating in the quietness of its cocoon, emerges as a butterfly. Whitmore (1991) suggests that transformation implies a movement from a negative state to a positive state. For this to occur a qualitative leap is required to effect a profound change. In archetypal mythology the mercurial god Hermes represents the mobile dynamic element within the transformative process. However, according to alchemical theory, the presence of a second element called the fixed is needed for change to be actualised. The goddess Hestia was known as Hermes' opposite and was said to contain the potential for fixation. The change itself usually happens as a result of an inner drive, but it is an additional ingredient that fixes the change. If transformation is not fixed, one of two things will happen: either the individual will be back at square one or the individual will find themselves in a state of constant disruption and disorder. In this chapter I would like to suggest that the fixing ingredient is critical reflection.

As an educationalist I am particularly interested in the teaching of reflective practice and have spent four years observing the transformation of novice nurses on their own voyage of discovery. Many travellers have embarked upon this journey. The personal testimonies which describe the hardships that individuals have experienced on the route to enlightenment and emancipation are demonstrated in this book (Fay 1987).

There seems to be an underlying purpose to these expressions, that of trying to create existential meaning out of personal experience. I am drawing here upon the philosophical beliefs of Kierkegaard (1944), whose theory hinges upon the fundamental assumption that only truths which are personally meaningful to the individual's life are of any relevance. And while there is angst in arriving at these personal truths,

Morrison (1992) suggests that man is not destroyed by this existential suffering; he is destroyed by suffering without meaning. It is this process of creating meaning out of suffering that I invite you to experience with me. For this journey the safety precautions are few but important. Firstly, it is important that you travel light. We are in search of soul – *all* that is needed here is your 'self'. Secondly, this story is my subjective truth. I say this not by way of an apology, but in the true existential manner. Really important truths are personal and like all such truths, this one needs to be approached with the greatest passion and sincerity. A journey that goes in search of soul begins with the goddess Psyche. Psyche was the Greek word for both 'soul' and 'butterfly', dating from the belief that human souls became butterflies while searching for a new reincarnation, a transformation.

Once, in a certain land, there dwelt a king and queen who had three daughters – the eldest charming for her bodily grace, the second equally charming for her wit and intelligence. Even as children everyone admired these two. But as time went on it began to be noised abroad that the third and youngest was after all the fairest of the three. The name of this one was Psyche. She was retiring, shy perhaps, nor had she all the gifts of her sisters; but it was seen that there was something unearthly in her beauty, some strange light in her countenance which entranced those who gazed upon it. Indeed it was whispered here and there that she was fairer than Aphrodite herself, whom all nature adores. And some, actually deserting the temples and the service of the foam born goddess, came and paid their worship to the lovely maiden.

Let us go in search of the goddess; leave the comfort of your temple and journey with me to the underworld. Learn to see in the dark, allow your eyes to become accustomed to the dimness and develop your capacity for night vision. I am here to serve you as an interpreter for the master workers – the alchemists. We join our travelling companion at the start of his journey in which he is searching. He comes across a fellow traveller along the way who is more experienced than he. Soon the two men become travelling companions and while they are journeying together the wiser man allows the younger and less experienced traveller to read some of his books to help the time pass. The young traveller enjoyed many books but as Coelho (1995) tells us, some carried special meaning:

> 'The book that most interested the boy told the stories of the famous alchemists. They were men who had dedicated their entire lives to the purification of metals in their dark underground laboratories; they believed that if a metal were heated for years, it would free itself of all its individual properties, and what was left would be the soul of the world. The soul of the world allowed them to understand anything on the face of the earth, because it was the language with which all things communicated. They called the discovery the master work – it was part liquid and part solid. The solid part was called the philosopher's

stone. The philosopher's stone had a fascinating property: a small sliver of the stone could transform large quantities of metal into gold. 'The boy asked of his friend, "can't you just observe men and omens in order to understand the language of alchemy?"

'Alchemy is a serious discipline; every step has to be followed exactly as it was followed by the masters. It's not so easy to find the philosopher's stone; the Englishmen spent years in their laboratories, observing the fire that purified the metals. They spent so much time close to the fire that gradually they gave up the vanities of the world. They discovered that a purification of the metals had led to a purification of themselves.' (Coelho 1995)

What is described here is the beginning of a journey for a novice, the new nurse, an apprenticeship which may last for many years, which although it may bring some sacrifices also brings a serendipity of other experiences. We are warned that we cannot learn by just watching the process, we have to be exposed to the journey ourselves. Kierkegaard (1944) suggests that it is only when we act and make significant choices that we relate to our own experience. It is essential to the transformative process that the individual nurse learns from her experience.

Socrates expounded that all true insight comes from within. This in itself is not an easy process. Bion (1974) said that people hate learning from experience. A person prefers to pick a ready-made suit off the shelf rather than make one for himself, even if it does not quite fit. Bion (1974) asserted that powerful forces operate in order to prevent us knowing what we truly think and feel. Instead we replace our own thoughts and feelings with substitutes. We are in the place of single vision, where the soul sleeps and appearances form themselves on the mind's eye like images on the photographic plate. In doing this I may speak another's ideas, thoughts and feelings about life, i.e. learning I have received (Belenky *et al.* 1986).

Alternatively I might take up the opposite posture and be determinedly against someone, his thoughts and ideas. Inherent in these assertions is not only the question of how do I become my subjective self, but also who is my subjective self. It seems that in order to travel along this road of transformation we need to take the risk of seeing ourselves as we truly are, coming to know ourselves through experience. But it does not stop there; fundamental questions will need to be faced. This, it seems, is a serious discipline in its own right, so much so that masters have outlined for us the steps which we are to follow closely if we are to experience the discovery of the philosopher's stone. One such master provides us with a map for locating the philosopher's stone. Poincare (1952) and Wallas (1926, cited in Neville 1989), upon analysing their own experiences, found that the journey could be broken down into four distinct stages:

(1)   An initial investigation termed the *preparation*
(2)   A period of rest known as the *incubation*

(3)   The occurrence of a sudden and *illuminatory* solution
(4)   Finally conscious rational development of understanding to validate the insight – *verification*

(Neville 1989).

The phase of preparation (how to turn metal into gold)

According to Neville (1989) the phase of preparation can be divided into
two distinct features. The first is to establish a data base out of which it is
hoped an insight will emerge. The second is to secure an appropriate
mental set. A clear element of that mental set must be, as already alluded
to, a batch of unanswered questions. These are not just any questions,
but questions that are existentially important to the individual – matters
of life that the traveller is intensely concerned with. In this place of two-
fold vision, the intellect is active and interest in appearances is scientific,
knowledge reigns and there exists intellectual knowing. Both the teacher
and the student need to stay in a place of uncertainty, prepared to
surrender to not knowing in order to create a transitional space for new
learning to occur.

What is the prima materia that prepares us for this long embarka-
tion? Some masters suggest one's ordinary everyday life experiences.
How is this so? If just ourselves and our own experiences seem little
preparation for a long and sometimes perilous journey, be reassured by
the words of Morenius, an old Arabic alchemist, who tells us that the
philosopher's stone is within us. Indeed it is described by Jung as our
archetypal self – the regulating centre of the psyche. But Morenius also
says that someone can find it in us – a special person who can see in us
what we cannot always see in ourselves. More recently reassurance has
come from a master who says that normal everyday experiences are
taken for granted and are therefore discarded along the way, but for-
tunately these may be seen within us by the super vision of another
(Johns 1995).

The period of incubation

' "I have known true alchemists," the more experienced traveller said.
"They locked themselves up in their dark laboratories and tried to
evolve, as gold had. And they found the philosopher's stone because
they understood that when something evolves, everything around
that thing evolves too. Others stumbled upon the stone by accident.
They already had the gift and their souls were readier for such things
than the souls of others. But these people are quite rare. And then
there were the others who were interested only in gold. They never
found the secret – anyone who interferes with destiny of another thing
never will discover his own.' (Coelho 1995)

This speaks to us of the challenge to our comfort zone, for surely true alchemists fall into the first category, being locked away in order to discover the regulating centre, walking blindly in the dark for a while until our eyes become accustomed to the shadows and the spectres become more familiar and less frightening. The soul indeed needs to be ready, for some are not yet open enough to be part of the discovery; and these souls cannot be rushed along, as Jung (1964) tells us that the philosopher's stone taken with the wrong attitude can also be deadly poison. Bion (1974) mirrors Jung's words when he writes of his belief that a thought has to emerge and cannot be forced into consciousness artificially. A good example of this is found in Ovid's ancient *Myth of Narcissus*. In this, the oldest version of the myth, Narcissus leant over the spring, enchanted by his own beauty, which he prided himself upon having the courage to admit. Narcissus admired his own reflection for so long that he became transfixed and died an early death. There is a significant division of the reflective episode into a stage of error and illusion and a stage of recognition and acknowledgment. Are these ancient masters saying that there is only one way to learn and that is through action – insight and experience? Indeed the wise amongst us recognise that the most significant learning is frequently accompanied or impelled by discomfort and tension (Joyce 1990).

Kierkegaard (1944) advocated that angst is positive. It is manifested in the individual who is actively engaged in an existential situation. Therefore angst may be the precursor to profound change. Yet we are also assured that incubation also means sleeping on it. Aldous Huxley (1994) describes his own incubation period as one of deep reflection which involved a sort of relaxed meditation. In this trance-like state he would let his thoughts happen to him and he is quoted as saying, 'I am thought, therefore I am'.

Bion (1974) has described this state as the presence of alpha functioning. He hypothesised that through alpha functioning, experiences are transformed into dream thoughts, personal possessions rather than mere facts. It is at this place of dynamic disequilibrium that the learning can take place – the attainment of personal truth – where the dark meets and is at once the same as the light. However, the fusion of the opposites which at their extremes tend to turn into one another, i.e. yin and yan, can also create a feeling of confusion. As the period of incubation reaches its climax and the philosopher's stone is awaiting its ascendance into the light, the tension mounts. It is at this point that the apprentice can feel compelled to force an early resolution, rather than bathe in the tension, waiting out the full incubation period.

Nursing theorists Newman (1986) and Parse (1987) suggest that it is the tension created by having to make choices throughout life, which pushes the nurse to higher levels of development. Further they suggest that higher levels of development, which may create tension and suffering, equate with expanding levels of creativity and improved caring. Awaiting the emerging purpose brings about a creative tension through which an expansion of consciousness can occur. In this phase it is essential for the nurse to develop what Keats called negative capability – the capacity to be with the uncertain:

> 'negative capability, that is, when a man is capable of being in uncertainties, mysteries, doubts, without any irritable reaching after fact and reason.' (Keats 1817, in Casement, 1985)

Illumination (the appearance of the gold)

The experience of deep relaxation does not only afford the individual more efficient processing and synthesising of data. The trance-like state that is induced in a state of reverie is the middle path trodden between the two opposites. This offers the opportunity of being in between worlds, having access to both the conscious and the unconscious, the right brain and the left brain. Bion (1974) suggests that the result of this reverie is a combination of an emotional and cognitive understanding – an intuitive understanding. From this intuitive understanding comes our three-fold vision, where the heart's knowledge is added to the mind's. In this space imagination is born.

Intuitive understanding, is often ascribed to the feminine, as is the soul. The feminine consciousness is the consciousness of Psyche, characterised by receptivity, inwardness, sensitivity and intuition. Enter the butterfly, Psyche, shy and retiring perhaps but her beauty is unearthly – not of this world. The type of consciousness that emerges out of the experience of Psyche is expanded consciousness or matriarchal consciousness, a consciousness that focuses around growth and transformation using the metaphors of conception (preparation), pregnancy (incubation) and birth (illumination). Miller and Miller (1994) state that:

> 'The knowledge revealed by the goddess is not one of learned or demonstrated truths, but a first hand experience of transformation. When your rational over-achieving ego-centred awareness has burnt out, your quiet, reflective lunar consciousness emerges to cool the fires of the spirit. The feminine holds the keys to experience of the inner planes for both men and women.' (p. 82)

This type of creative illuminative thinking is a very ordinary and everyday operation, but it generally emerges as knowledge without any awareness of the process; the period of incubation is taken for granted or cut short. What happens to this newly formed nugget of gold?

> ' "This is why alchemy exists," said the boy, "so that everyone will search for treasure, find it and then want to be better than he was in his former life. That's what alchemists do, they show you that when we strive to be better than we are, everything around us becomes better too. It is we who nourish the soul of the world, and the world we live in will be either better or worse, depending on whether we become better or worse".' (Coelho 1995)

We discover here that enlightenment of our own path leads the way to further paths. But we also learn that when we seek out our own light and shine it, it actually helps illuminate the path for others to see their way. However, just as the bright light casts a shadow, so our own light will also illuminate our own and other people's shadows. The epicentre of the earthquake is so strong that its ripples are felt for miles around. Yet the illumination, powerful as it is, is like the striking of a match, a momentary experience and the difficult and sometimes tedious process of discovery must start again. How do we know where, when and how to begin? Perhaps the answer is to begin where we end – truly unifying our experience of the opposites.

Verification (beginning or end?)

How do we differentiate between the generation of new ideas, pre-paration, from their evaluation – verification. At which point are we actively engaged in the doing and when are we being inactive? These two phases are as often ignored in the creation of ideas and experiences as the phases of incubation and illumination are taken for granted. The liquid and the solid parts of the philosopher's stone are symbolic of this schism. And yet without either the art or science, we would have no knowledge of the other.

It is pointless to argue that one method of verification is better than the other. As in the illumination phase, we need to recognise the importance of both, unifying the perceived opposites to create a third eye. Many travellers have spoken about the vision of the third eye, gained from treading the middle path (Jung 1964). Kierkegaard (1944) also addressed this in his writings relating to life forms. He described three stages, the two lower stages being the aesthetic and the ethical. The aesthetic person has a reflective attitude to reality, living for the moment, whereas the ethical person is serious, dedicated and consistent in nature, concerned with moral choices. As you can see, one is as important as the other, the first offering us the ability to reflect-in-action, the second affording the opportunity to reflect-on-action (Schön 1987).

Neville (1989) stresses the importance of paying attention to the subtle signals in our whole organism, not just those of our intellect or of our feelings. By paying attention to our corporeal and ethereal responses we become more deeply connected to our authentic self. This type of deeply personal experience is sometime referred to as tacit knowledge. Thus we can respond from a place of congruence, the match between what I think and feel, what I say and what I do, a position of faith in my personal truth. This takes us to Kierkegaard's third stage, the religious stage of faith, faith in self and others. The experience of four-fold vision may be felt as spiritual insight, the power to perceive divine reality. When the imagination has finished its work and the actions of the senses are synthesised, the soul reigns triumphant.

'The more experienced traveller lit the fire and placed some lead in the iron pan. When the lead had become liquid, the alchemist took from his pouch the strange yellow egg. He scraped from it a sliver as thin as hair, wrapped it in wax and added it to the pan. When the pan had cooled the boy looked at it dazzled. The lead had turned into gold. "Will I learn to do that someday?" the boy asked.

"This was my destiny not yours," the traveller answered, "but I wanted to show you that it was possible.' (Coelho 1995).

As our journey comes to its end, I can only verify my truth in the moment, that truth may change as soon as this chapter is written, it may even be changing as I am formulating my ideas. After all, personal truth is not the end of the journey, it is only the beginning. The journey will be changed as a result of exposure to new experiences, but then that is what makes my life meaningful. In the creation of meaning my contribution may be helpful, but it may be neither necessary nor sufficient. Meaning is Psyche's work. It is the depth in things which Psyche must search out, soul seeking soul.

References

Belenky, M., Clinchy, B., Goldberger, N. & Tarule, J. (1986) *Women's Ways of Knowing* Basic Books, New York.

Bion, W. (1974) *Bion's Brazilian lectures*, vol. 2. Imago editoria, Rio de Janeiro.

Casement, P. (1985) *On Learning from the Patient*. Routledge, London.

Coelho, P. (1995) *The Alchemist*. Thorsons, London.

Fay, B. (1987) *Critical Social Science*. Polity Press, Cambridge.

Huxley, A. (1994) *The Human Situation*. Flamingo, London.

Jacoby, M. (1990) *Individuation and Narcissism*. Routledge, London.

Johns, C. (1995) The value of reflective practice for nursing. *Journal of Clinical Nursing*, **4**(1), 23–30.

Joyce, B.R. (1990) Dynamic disequilibrium: the intelligence of growth. *Theory into Practice*. **xxiii**(1), 26–34.

Jung, C. (1964) *Man and his Symbols*. Picador, London.

Kierkegaard, S. (1944) *The Concept of Dread*. Princeton University Press, New Jersey.

Miller, R. & Miller, I. (1994) *The Modern Alchemists*. Phanes Press, USA.

Morrison, R. (1992) Diagnosing spiritual pain in patients. *Nursing Standard*, **6**(25), 36–8.

Neville, B. (1989) *Educating Psyche*. Collins, Victoria.

Newman, M. (1986) *Health as Expanding Consciousness*. Mosby, St Louis.

Parse, R.R. (1987) *Nursing Science: Major Paradigms, Theories and critiques*. Saunders, Philadelphia.

Schön, D. (1987) *Educating the Reflective Practitioner*. Josey Bass, San Francisco.

Whitmore, D. (1991) *Psychosynthesis Counselling in Action*. Sage, London.

Chapter 15
The Reflective Journey Begins a Spiritual Journey

Stephen Wright

Introduction

The central aim of reflective practice is to help nurses increase awareness of their practice and to develop it further to improve the quality of patient care. Much of the literature on the theme has focused on this principal purpose, and yet there may be other dimensions worthy of consideration. There is a tendency in nursing to view issues in isolation, assuming a linear cause–effect relationship between nurse and practice. For example, a nurse learns about primary nursing, develops it in practice, and care is changed in some way. Likewise, reflective practice, often twinned with the concept of clinical supervision, is assumed to produce a similar cause–effect phenomenon. However, if a more holistic view is taken, such a paradigm may seem somewhat limited and reductionist. Thus it can be argued that nurses as human beings, in all their infinite complexity in an infinitely complex universe, are unlikely to respond to any issue in a simple way. For example, developing an area of nursing practice – whether it be primary nursing, participating in an educational programme, or working in a developing team – whatever the cause, it seems possible to argue that a transformation in nursing practice will bring with it a transformation in the nurse.

Changing nurses and nursing in parallel is not a new phenomenon (Salvage & Wright 1995). The assumption that each is inextricably linked with the other has underpinned much of the work of the nursing development unit movement. Nurses do not don their roles at work and act as if isolated from the essence of themselves as persons. That which affects and informs us as nurses spills over into our thinking and behaviour in the wider world and vice versa. We do not stand hermetically sealed in the various roles we occupy in our lives; each flows into and affects and is affected by the other.

Thus what follows in this chapter is a discussion on how reflective practice may not only concern the transformation of practice, but also the transformation of the nurse, and the nurse as a person in all her many facets in the world cannot be untouched by what happens in one part of that world. The part is affected by the whole, the whole affected by the part.

Furthermore, some phenomena in nursing may have a more powerful effect on personal transformation than others. Some issues may produce radical effects upon personal awareness and ways of being in the world, while others may seem at first sight to leave us relatively untouched – like the difference between missing a bus or surviving a serious accident. Likewise no two persons can be expected to respond to outwardly similar phenomena in the same way. I have worked with groups of nurses in the practice of meditation. A group subject to the same meditation technique may produce individual responses as diverse as nothing particular of note through to awareness of anxiety, or deep relaxation to profound spiritual experiences. Thus reflective practice may have ramifications beyond changing nursing practice. As an instrument of inner work, it may vary in its effects from changing the way we work to the way we see ourselves in the world and the greater realm of being.

Spirituality and religion

When considering the spiritual dimensions of reflective practice, are these necessarily the same as religious dimensions? The two terms, religion and spirituality, are often used interchangeably; yet while being closely related they are quite different. Religion is seen by Artress (1995) as the form or structure given to the expression of certain beliefs, usually acted out collectively. A religion serves to provide a community with a sense of common purpose and shared values and actions, and a safe framework to explore the nature of our spirituality and relationship to the divine.

> 'Religion is the outward form, the 'container', specifically the liturgy and all the acts of worship that teach, praise, and give thanks to God.' (Artress 1995)

Spirituality can be seen as that for which religion is the 'container', the inward activity of growth and maturation that brings us to an understanding of who we are, our purpose and our relationship to that which is greater than ourselves. Stoter (1995) sees spirituality as:

> 'the total personality which links aspects together, expressed through relationships, personal practices and beliefs. It enables the search for meaning in life and provides a common bond between individuals'.

For some people, it may be a deepening of their humanistic values and awareness of the self in relation to the wider world, and may not necessarily include acceptance of God. However, many have argued (Schumacher 1978; Jones 1994, Artress 1995; Vaughan 1995) that an inner exploration of the self leads not only to a deeper relationship with the self, but also a growing acceptance of the divinity that pervades everything.

Challenging the view that 'this is all there is', Schumacher (1978) believes that:

> 'if the great cosmos is seen as nothing but a chaos of particles without purpose or meaning, so man must be seen as nothing but a chaos of particles without purpose and meaning – a sensitive chaos, indeed, capable of suffering pain, anguish and despair, but a chaos all the same... a rather unfortunate cosmic accident of no consequence whatsoever.'

He goes on to suggest that a person fixed entirely on:

> 'the philosophy of materialistic scientism, denying the reality of the "invisibles" and confining his attention solely to what can be counted, measured and weighed , lives in a very poor world, so poor that he will experience it as a meaningless wasteland unfit for human habitation. Equally, if he sees it as nothing but an accidental collocation of atoms he will needs agree with Bertrand Russell that the only rational attitude is one of "unyielding despair".'

Jones (1994) argues that the 'goal of childhood is to separate, the goal of adulthood is to connect' and this connection is clearly beyond an understanding of 'who I am', rather 'a rediscovery of those experiences of connection to a reality beyond the ordinary world of space and time that gives our life meaning and purpose'. Those experiences have often been lost in modern culture, with its emphasis upon inidividualist materialism and religion as ritual; experience without meaning. Indeed, it has been argued that the obsession with form and ritual causes many people to turn away from the organised religions, because the organisation itself inhibits the inner exploration which can lead to a personal connection with God; while religions have tended for many reasons, among them the fear of the risks associated with an individual mystical path, to emphasise conformity to established doctrine and practice.

Jones goes on to argue that 'a vital and growing spirituality may depend more on the recovery of a vital and growing selfhood than on the revival of any particular religious forms' and that 'spirituality is both a theory and a practice. The word experiment and experience have the same root. Spirituality says, do certain things and you will experience your connection with the sacred'. However, if organised religions can, for some, inhibit rather than promote that personal search and connection, then the spiritual search may remain unsatisfied. Artress (1995) believes that this loss of the personal experience of the mystical connection with the divine lies at the root of the malaise in and disaffection from many religions. She suggests that:

> 'Christianity lost its meaning and its power to transform lives when it threw out its mystical teachings. The inner way seemed dangerous

and complicated. That is why there has been so much emphasis on the Transcendent God, who is perceived as outside ourselves. Both aspects of God are important, but we have created a religious ideology that values one to the exclusion of the other, and is therefore incomplete.'

This theme is echoed by Fox (1983) who supports:

'the rich theme of creation centred spirituality of humankind's divinization. While Eastern Christianity never lost this theme in its theology, the West struggled to keep it alive after the all pervading influence of Augustine's guilty conscience reduced salvation to cleansing from sin instead of awakening to divine potential, divine beauty.'

Thus there is the possibility that a spiritual journey may be pursued through personal inner work as well as, perhaps even separate from, the constraints of organised religion. But how is this opening to be achieved and does not such a journey carry risks?

Many authors, both ancient and new, acknowledge the risks of pursuing a spiritual journey without guidance and the protection provided by religious forms of practice. However, it is precisely these restraints which may inhibit the journey for some, while providing a safe space for exploration for others. From the Sufi approach to Islam as illuminated in Farud ud-Din Attar's 12th century *Conference of the Birds* (Darbandi & Davis 1984), or Christian mysticism such as *The Dark Night of the Soul* (St John of the Cross, trans. Zimmerman 1907), or *The Cloud of Unknowing* (author unknown, trans. Wolters 1961), to the Hindu and Buddhist spiritual traditions, all speak of the risks to the self of an unsupported and unguided spiritual path. Storr (1996) warns against the entrapments of cults and gurus, while Vaughan (1995) recalls that the individualised 'pick and mix' approach is equally risky in its lack of discipline, focus and direction. It seems that guidance is necessary, but Storr (1996) believes this guidance should come from those who empower and encourage us along the path, rather than seeking to control and dominate to bring the spiritual traveller under the power of the guide. Jones (1995) in accepting the risks involved writes:

'The question of finding a spiritual path becomes, in part, "to what can I give myself unreservedly?". Dangerous? Yes, but especially dangerous is a life without ecstasy, without the numinous, without depth, breadth, passion, meaning or purpose. Spirituality is process before content. Not memorising rules, facts or concepts, but freeing the mind and the heart to explore new worlds of insight.'

For many such authors throughout history, it seems that the spiritual journey, despite its risks, cannot be avoided.

Nurses and spirituality

A full debate on the nature of spirituality is beyond the scope of this chapter, but it can be deduced from the above discussion that the desire for a deeper connection and awakening is present in everyone, and nurses do not exist in encapsulated or isolated roles. Latterly it has been argued (Bradshaw 1994) that nursing, in the wake of the influence of humanistic theories applied through nursing models, has lost its sense of direction. Stoter (1995) believes that the spiritual care of patients has become something that nurses have increasingly ignored, or reduced to equating it to religious care. He writes that 'to see spiritual care only as religious care limits its true nature and tends to relegate it to a footnote at the end of the ward report, or something to be handed on to another professional. Thus nurses seem to have turned away from a whole area of care that is significant to patients.' One possible cause might be, as Snow and Willard's study (1989) suggests, that nurses cannot support patients appropriately with their spiritual needs simply because they themselves are denying its significance in their own lives. Thus

> 'Without faith in a power greater than ourselves – greater than our parents – we have difficulty with relationships that operate on other than surface levels. We often are afraid to be honest with ourselves or to believe in the honesty of another's love. Further, without spirituality, we find it impossible to believe in something better for ourselves. The cynical messages – from society, or families, our colleagues, our friends – that tell us to settle for less than trust, honesty, and intimacy in relationships nourish the delusion that we can't have a relationship on a deep level... A relationship without spirituality is a frightening place to be. Spirituality assures us we are not alone. Spirituality assures us we do not have to be in control of others, what they do, what they feel, what they think. Spirituality gives us the courage to trust, to be honest and, therefore, vulnerable, and to live in acceptance of ourselves and others.'

Barnum (1996) echoes these concerns and argues that before nurses can fully care for others, they must also care for themselves; connecting in relationship to others also requires that nurses connect at a deeper level with themselves.

The impact on nursing of spiritual disconnection produces a deep malaise, affecting not only the quality of patient care, but exacerbating demoralisation, disaffection, and a whole range of illnesses among nurses. This 'soul sickness' (Moore 1992) can pervade all aspects of our lives, but may itself be a catalyst for change when we become aware of its impact upon us.

Opening the gate – reflective practice as a portal for transformation

As part of an ongoing study looking at spirituality in nursing, several nurses I interviewed began to indicate that reflection on and in their practice was having an impact that transcended changes in their day to day work.

> **Rosemary:** Each time I met with my (clinical) supervisor we talked about the usual stuff, but we always seemed to end up talking about the way I was feeling. I know I am doing a good job, I know I am, but something seems to be missing. I can't put my finger on it, a sort of hopelessness or emptiness. I seem to be working my socks off every day, but just not feeling right. You know what I mean? There's more, there has to be more than this drudge. I'm caring, but at the end of the day, who's caring for me. I mean, I just keep feeling what's the point, why am I doing this. There has to be more to it than the pay-packet or the chance that a patient will be grateful for what I do.

Rosemary's situation seems to reflect that loss of purpose and the sense of powerlessness which Snow and Willard (1989) attribute to the need for a deeper meaning and connection with our work. One nurse found that working with her tutor on a module of training for therapeutic touch (TT) meant having to question long cherished beliefs about himself and the nature of his relationships with his patients.

> **Geoff:** As the months went by I began to think 'this really works,' but it made me realise that I was not who I thought I was. Accepting that something I was somewhat sceptical about actually worked, that I could do it, turned my world upside down. After each talk with my teacher, when we went through my diary, I could feel myself opening up. It sounds daft to say it, but I felt myself changing, new ideas and new worlds were opening up before me. I was never told, this is the way it is, this is what you have to do; rather, it seemed like a gentle feeding – try this book, listen to this music and so on – that's the way it's happened for me. Now I can't read enough, and sometimes I feel like I'm becoming a different person as well as a different nurse.

Another nurse working in the community illustrates the impact of caring for a particular patient and how she worked through her experiences with a colleague. In this case there was no formal clinical supervisory relationship, just a supportive workmate who would sit and listen to her about her experiences, acting as a mirror reflecting back what she saw as her colleague's needs and actions.

> **Pam:** It got worse each day, entering the house knowing he was there and that he would be worse than the day before. I knew what I was doing was O.K. but that didn't remove the feeling of helplessness. In the face of his pain, his suffering, once the drugs were done there was nothing, nothing I could do or say; it had all been done and said. So I would just sit there, hold his hand a little maybe, listen to his stories, and in the end I had to leave him to that

lonely house. And I thought, God keep me from dying like this, alone and friendless, and I'd feel awful every day I left, you know, every day, it would just hang around me. I've nursed hundreds far worse than him, but he got to me for some reason, really got to me. My husband used to get angry, told me to leave the job if I couldn't cope. It was Pat (colleague) who kept me sane. I hadn't realised how much it was me that was dying with that man, how he showed me one of my deepest terrors. I began to realise what a cold fish I'd become at work until I met him, treating death matter of factly like another dressing or injection. I eventually went to a therapist for a while and I've found myself being drawn back to church again. It feels good to be there, but I've never been taken with all the fuss and talk and hymns and things like that. I like the quietness, sometimes I go on my own and just sit and listen ... the stillness, sometimes so still you can feel it ...

Perhaps Pam's story illustrates Stoter's (1995) comment that:

'to be opening oneself to pain and suffering, to the sufferer's beliefs and to a patient's or family's search for meaning in life inevitably brings exposure to the carer's own beliefs. An essential part of resourcing for carers is to examine regularly their own values and beliefs, and to identify what they feel is important for themselves.'

If Snow and Willard (1989) and others are correct in their assertion that there is a great longing in nursing for nurses to connect more deeply with themselves and their patients, then there is a need to examine what contexts can be created for this to be done safely and lovingly. Spirituality seems to be little more than a footnote in modern nursing education, and many nurses, if the endless media reports and surveys of declining morale and rising workloads are accepted, find it difficult in the everyday workworld to find the space to explore what has heart and meaning for them. Increasing competitiveness in organisations, the emphasis on outcomes rather than processes at work, and the adherence to the age old belief that nurses must always 'cope' (Salvage 1986) – all these factors and more conspire to inhibit spiritual exploration by nurses. In such a world, even those who wish to take the first tentative steps may find themselves held back by the majority who deny such needs.

However, as the above examples appear to illustrate, there are many ways in which a spiritual awakening can be nourished. Currently, many authors in the field have noted how psychotherapy is filling the gap left behind by the formal religions (Jones 1994; Artress 1995; Vaughan 1995) in terms of providing the context for an exploration of such matters, as well as noting the enormous numbers of people who are turning to alternative 'new age' approaches, be they ancient techniques such as shamanism or the myriad mystical pathways which seem to be on offer in an extensive range of journals and courses.

Reflective practice could hardly lay claim to being a spiritual discipline, but it does seem to hold the potential for some nurses to act as a gateway for a more intimate journey into who we are and what place we hold in the scheme of things. However small the gate may seem, and however small the steps may be that are taken through it, perhaps it is possible that one more avenue is available to us to begin or continue that inner work. 'Probing our own spirit always brings humans to the border of spirit in its larger sense' (Chopra 1993). Reflective practice seems to offer one model in which that probing may occur.

If it is accepted that the reflective journey may also stimulate a spiritual journey, then it is clear that more work needs to be done to clarify what support mechanisms need to be in place to ensure that it is done safely. What skills and attributes does a clinical supervisor need in order to know when someone is in spiritual need and when to help? How do we know when to guide the person on to other means of support and what and who are those other supports? The many questions such as these seem thus far to have been largely avoided in the collective body of nursing. At best, a referral to the appropriate minister is often all that has been suggested until recently – whether it is a patient or nurse who is in need. More recently, the new 'high priests' – the counsellors and therapists – seem to have usurped them.

The questions beg further study, and the work of authors such as Snow and Willard (1989) and Barnum (1996) appear to be offering a number of ways forward, not least in raising the profile of the significance of spirituality to the future of nursing and nurses. It is more than an issue of the quality of care or education. Reflective practice seems to offer a step, perhaps a first step for some, into a greater realm of being, and as Artress (1995) again reminds us:

'If you have gone deeply within yourself and experienced mystery of your being, the mystery of God reveals itself. Knowing the depths of our being, both the shadow and the light, introduces us to the vastness of the Spirit, the Sacred held within each of us.'

References

Artress, L. (1995) *Walking a Sacred Path*. Riverhead, New York.

Darbandi, A. & Davis, D. (1984) *The Conference of the Birds*. Translated from the twelfth century original by Farud ud-Din Altar. Penguin, Harmondsworth.

Barnum, B. (1996) *Spirituality in Nursing – from Tradition to New Age*. Springer, New York.

Bradshaw, A. (1994) *Lighting the Lamp – the Spiritual Dimension of Nursing Care*. Scutari, Harrow.

Chopra, D. (1993) *Ageless Body; Timeless Mind*. Crown, London.

Fox, M. (1983) Julian's contribution to spiritual needs today. In *Meditations with Julian of Norwich* (B. Doyle). Bear, Santa Fe.

Jones, J. (1994) *In the Middle of This Road We Call Our Life*. Harper Collins, London.

Moore, T. (1992) *Care of the Soul*. Piatkus, London.

Salvage, J. (1986) *The Politics of Nursing*. Heinemann, London.

Salvage, J. & Wright, S.G. (1995) *Nursing Development Units*. Scutari, Harrow.

Schumacher, E.F. (1978) *A Guide for the Perplexed*. Abacus, London.

Snow, C. & Willard, P. (1989) *I'm Dying to Take Care of You*. Professional Counsellor Books, Redmond, NJ.

St John of the Cross, Trans. Zimmerman Rev. B. (1907) *The Dark Night of the Soul*. Clarke, Cambridge.

Storr, A. (1996) *Feet of Clay*. HarperCollins, London.

Stoter, D. (1995) *Spiritual Aspects of Health Care*. Mosby, London.

Vaughan, F. (1995) *Shadows of the Sacred*. Quest, Wheaton, Illinois.

Wolters, C. (1961) Trans. from the original, author unknown. *The Cloud of Unknowing*. Penguin, Harmondsworth.

Chapter 16

The Supervisor's Story: from Expert to Novice

Jan Bailey

Introduction

The journey involved in compiling this chapter has been both evocative and enlightening. It begins with some reflective snapshots of my early life and represents my largely uncontrived use of reflective thoughts, feelings and actions. This provides a backdrop for the recording of some significant moments from my practice as a mental health nurse and unqualified nurse teacher, which were perhaps pivotal in propelling me forward onto new paths which I did not yet know. I was largely resistant for many years to the conscious use of reflection in my personal and professional life. I perceived the reflective path to be one in which I had already walked, as though reflection had some definitive end point.

It was not until I returned to education, when learning to teach, that I began to truly embrace reflection and reflective practice as more than a slogan for practice. The stories taken from my student teacher days exemplify this transformation in my personal and professional life. On reflection, I remember feeling a mixture of excitement and anxiety, because the reflective path felt as though I were walking on shifting sand. I hope that the readers of this chapter and indeed the whole book will be encouraged and challenged to tell their own stories of reflective journeys and give voice to one of the most significant developments in nursing and nurse education: reflective practice.

Walking down the same path: personal transformation

I was born the second daughter of a working class Lancashire family of six. Following an unremarkable and controlled childhood I emerged as a troubled and challenging adolescent, which created friction, tension and turbulence with my parents. I felt powerless in my position, unable to communicate effectively or to negotiate compromises with my parents. I turned to music, art and the performing arts as ways in which to express my feelings. At this time I discovered musicians and artists who appeared to be conveying similar turbulence and conflict with life, the most significant and notable for me being the poet and singer Leonard Cohen (1975, 1992) and the graphic artist M.C. Escher (1989). Cohen expressed through his lyrics the same anguish, angst and despair that I often felt and, although many have described his music as 'songs to commit suicide to', I felt hope that there were others who doubted and questioned the human condition as I did.

Escher also offered me hope. His graphic work depicted a vision of other worlds, other possibilities, other questions and other answers. The impossible etchings which he produced offered me insight into the chaos of the reality in which I found myself as a teenager. I viewed Escher, like Cohen, as kindred and reassuring spirits. My despair was felt by others who had found a way to articulate those emotions through the medium of music and art work. This realisation helped me develop my own artistic and creative pursuits as methods of expression which were safer than confrontations with authority figures and relatively free from the interference of anyone.

Despite this, or perhaps because of this, I left school at the earliest opportunity. I didn't enjoy my grammar school education, I never really thought I fitted in. In retrospect I can now see that I didn't understand the middle class educational system in which I was unlucky enough to have gained a place. I struggled with academic work, the culture and function of the school and differences in language, which Bernstein (1975) acknowledged in his work on social class. A classic 'school failure' I triumphantly left school at 16, without academic qualifications and blissfully unaware that I was destined to a series of dull, monotonous factory employments. My priority was economic and personal independence; my need to leave home superseded any thoughts of a career.

After three years of factory work and still at home, but engaged now to a working class man, I realised that I was in danger of continuing to walk down the same path as my parents walked. I passed the nursing entrance test and embarked on what was to become my nursing career. My fiance issued an ultimatum in response to the changes which I was experiencing due to my nursing course, which for me were exciting but for him intolerable. I chose my career.

It was for very mixed reasons then, that I became a psychiatric nurse. In part I wanted to help and understand others in emotional distress, and partly to help myself gain insight into my own emotional problems. My career was successful and I learned and practised my craft in a variety of settings spanning the public and private healthcare sectors. Through the years I spent several periods in personal psychotherapy, which resolved childhood issues and helped me as a person and a professional (Paterson & Zderad 1976). I also served as a nurse in the Armed Services for a short period, but due to my lack of military discipline (I was too challenging and questioning to ever make a 'good' soldier), I left to take up further nurse training. After a further five years of clinical practice I experienced what has come to be known as 'burnout' and also felt disatisfied with my membership of what I perceived to be an unchanging and undervalued semi-profession.

Although I was considered an effective mental health practitioner, I often felt that I was just going through the motions at work and this worried me. Perhaps more worryingly, it seemed to me that many of my colleagues who had been nursing longer than me were similarly just going through the motions, but had ceased to worry about it. There were other issues too. I had always considered that one of the main attributes of an effective mental health practitioner was to be an excellent communicator, in particular to possess and practise expert listening skills as well as a genuine desire to be with patients in distress. I perceived that in contrast to my views the most experienced nurses often had the least contact with patients.

Despite administration and management tasks I found that I was able to spend at least 90% of my working shift with patients. Some of my colleagues seemed to emerge from the office only to dispense drugs and seemed reluctant to engage with clinical work. Also, I had noticed that some nursing staff appeared to have mastered the art of talking to patients, but seemed unwilling or unable to listen, to use silence effectively, or just be with patients.

Although a school failure, with only nursing qualifications which were unrecognised for accreditation in universities 10 years ago, I enrolled on a part-time certificate course at a local university. When I passed this I gained more confidence in my self and also now possessed the academic wherewithal to pursue undergraduate studies, in order to get myself a 'proper job'. I had decided to focus on political and social studies for my degree, intending to totally veer away from all things nursing. On reflection, I can now see that the two subjects I took at university were actually closely interelated with my experiences as a nurse, more of a natural progression rather than a real change of direction.

I found academic work this time round a totally positive experience, almost diametrically opposite to my schooling. The degree was stimulating and challenging in ways which were unexpected, which reflects for me as a teacher the spontaneity and unpredictability of the learning process. I gradually learned how to read academic texts and found that although I could read a novel in a night, I could only read one or two pages of an academic text before needing a rest. With persistence this improved and soon I was reading texts related and unrelated to my degree studies.

My education which I intended to be a means to an end, i.e. get a degree and then a 'proper job', had changed and become education as an end in itself. My politics tutors used to joke with me that I could probably have got another degree in literature. This was because I had read many Russian and Japanese novels in an attempt to understand the nature and culture of these people as a prelude to understanding the politics of both countries. My experiences as a person, through insights and resolutions in therapy, my practice as a nurse and my educational endeavours, combined to effect my personal transformation.

Walking down another path: professional transformation

I commenced a full-time initial teacher preparation course, following two highly enjoyable and fulfilling years as an apprentice teacher in a college of nursing. To some extent I continued to walk down the same path as before. For example, I believed that I was already a competent teacher and I was able to sustain this belief through two thirds of the course, despite challenges from several sources to the contrary. A highly emotive interview with the course leader following my referral on two of the course modules proved to be a critical turning point and the beginning of my professional transformation.

My eyes became open to the reality of both my academic and practice shortcomings and the exposure of my belief and value systems which perpetuated my distorted perceptions. In beginning to unravel these processes of insight, challenge and change I began to articulate my transformation. The following passages represent some of my attempts to chart this development through reflective writing in my student teacher experiences and as a nurse educator.

Stories from student days

Unfreezing and dipping my toes in the water of reflection

I came to the course with the belief that I was already a competent teacher. This was based on my previous experiences of teaching practice. Also, I came to the course with fixed expectations of my role as a student, believing that I would receive from experts the required academic knowledge to assimilate and then reproduce in order to pass the course. My fixed and blinkered thinking and actions were very apparent in my educational practice. For example, I limited student evaluation of my teaching practice to collecting data on the process skills of teaching, which I already knew I was proficient at. By doing this I was resisting exposure of my weaknesses and avoiding any real critique of my practice. I was stuck or frozen, fearful of gaining 'negative' feedback, but unable to shift, develop or grow because of my reluctance to seek out meaningful evaluation.

My anxiety levels were high as I began to realise how disorganised and unknowledgeable I was. My teaching practice was based on my abilities to deliver content in humorous and creative ways and totally lacked any considerations of teaching and learning theories and how they could be used, refined and developed in practice. This was exposed by the course leader on several occasions, but my psychological barriers and habitual thinking resisted this exposure. Instead I sought and received positive feedback from other experienced teachers and students which reinforced my beliefs about my competence as a teacher. I continued not to plan teaching sessions in systematic or rigorous ways. I was relatively blind and unable to see the many gaping holes in my practice and knowledge base.

Following the incident with the course leader, I began to experience some conflict and doubt about our different perceptions of my competence and development. I became open to her interpretation of reality and caught glimpses of myself through her eyes. I began to expose my fears and anxieties and the limitations of my practice to myself and others and felt enormous relief that I no longer had to pretend that my practice was perfect. Once I had accepted and articulated this, I was able to begin to change and develop my practice. I gained tremendous support from peers and tutors who commented on and therefore validated the dramatic changes which I was undergoing, and this gave me more confidence to develop my skills and knowledge. I have become reflective and found a new way of being in life and in professional practice. I can never return to being an unknowing, blinkered person or practitioner. Reflection and the gaining of insight cannot be unknown once they are known.

Challenging beliefs and values through reflection on action

Now that the unfreezing stage has begun and I am emerging from the ice of my blinkered thinking, I am developing insights into my relationships with others in professional practice. An example of this is a realisation that despite my claim to be humanistic in my practice, I actually perceive students in quite traditional ways. The reality of my practice does not fit or match my espoused theory and this has come as somewhat of a shock to me. I doubt and challenge the reality and efficacy of my thoughts, feelings and actions, and can trace the background and causes of my habitual practice to my apprenticeship teaching years.

These habits have become internalised beliefs, which have become part of my teacher practice. One of these beliefs is my continued use of confrontation with students who talk in class. I unconsciously viewed this behaviour as disrespectful and often labelled such students 'difficult'. In unravelling this label that I apply to students I have learned that this reveals more about my own educational values, beliefs and power relationships than it does about student behaviour. For example, what do I mean by difficult? Difficult for whom? Perhaps I make these judgements because I'm feeling threatened and self-conscious and also so I don't have to look too closely at my own practice.

In reality, I have no knowledge of why students may talk in class but I tend to take a negative view of this, hence my confrontational response when it occurs. It may be that students are sharing their views because they are interested in the session. Perhaps they are bored because I've pitched the session at the wrong level. There could be all sorts of reasons why students talk in class, but my labelling them as 'difficult' and confronting them, does not help to further my understanding of their behaviour or facilitate and promote an effective learning environment. My strategy of confrontation is very risky and may belittle or anger the student it is directed at – hardly an example of humanistic practice on my part.

Instead, I have realised that making judgements such as these, based on little or no knowledge of student behaviour, is indicative of my own habitual thinking and practices. It centres around my expectations of acceptable and unacceptable student behaviour, based on ideas about myself as teacher in control and in authority in the classroom. To overcome this, I have started to use my feelings, thoughts and actions in open and honest ways with students and others. In teaching practice my use of self and the exposure of my feelings appears to better facilitate a teaching and learning partnership. Once this is established I can really negotiate teaching sessions with students to achieve student centred learning; by building in appropriate periods of reflection and interaction, students are enabled to express their needs and feelings.

By uncovering these issues of control and power in the classroom, I have been able to reflect on and subsequently change my teacher beliefs, thinking and actions. Consequently, now if students talk in class I rarely view this as a negative phenomenon, although it still challenges my practice. Instead, I ignore the behaviour and have found that students themselves control disruption to their learning very positively, which reflects the effectiveness of peer group pressure. The adoption of less negative and non-judgemental approaches to teaching and learning fits better with my espoused humanistic approaches.

The following reflection is taken from my ongoing educational prac-tice. Once I had completed my teaching course, I returned to my former college of nursing as a qualified and presumably competent teacher. My return to the organisation posed huge problems for me. Like many returning teachers, I fell into the trap of attempting to fill up my empty diary with as much teaching as I could, to the point of overload. I was desperately trying to seek out a new role for myself, to reflect the changes which I had and still was experiencing. Because I had become reflective and was changing so much I experienced a huge culture shock on return to my former workplace.

I felt that I didn't speak the same language as some of my colleagues. My enthusiasm to share my reflective stories of teacher practice, lifelong learning and portfolio development was not always understood or well received. On the other hand, there were others who wanted to know more, particularly students, student teachers and some of my colleagues who were developing reflective practice in clinical areas. I learned to share my stories more effectively with those willing to listen and was rewarded with hearing their stories develop and unfold. In this way I learned to survive as a changed person and practitioner, in what I perceived was a largely unchanged organisation.

A teaching and learning story

I received my feedback today about a teaching session in which I was peer reviewed by a colleague. It was disappointing because the session occurred over a month ago and we have only just got together to discuss it. The memories of the event have faded for myself and the reviewer somewhat and I have realised how important it is to get feedback straight away. It was useful that I had critiqued myself directly afterwards and got excellent feedback from students, which I had written up in my reflective diary. We discussed the session and I refreshed both our memories by using these written accounts. A number of interesting and surprising issues concerning teaching and reflection arose from our discussion, which made me realise several things.

It is crucial to receive verbal feedback and desirable to receive written feedback immediately after the event has occurred. This is important for me as I am constantly aiming to improve my practice by improving my skills and knowledge about teaching and learning and by testing out various theoretical educational perspectives in action. Receiving feedback so long after the event meant that the points raised were less meaningful and 'alive'. Valuable comments about the negative and positive aspects of my practice are less accessible to both of us and the delay means that I am unable to act upon the feedback immediately to improve my future performances.

I was reminded of my advice to students about the importance of recording reflections as soon as possible after an incident has occurred or risk forgetting and omitting valuable emotional and situational data, making the reflection less meaningful. Others, such as Boud *et al.* (1985) acknowledge the importance of writing reflective notes for the later and central goal of reconstructing experience, in order to make the experience meaningful. My reviewer had no written notes on the event, which hampered the potential for us both to learn and reflect on the experience in a meaningful way.

The quality of the feedback is also dependent on the skills, knowledge and reflective capacity of the reviewee and reviewer. I found in this session that the comments made by the reviewer were unfocused, general and unconnected to any theoretical considerations. This was another disappointment as I had asked her to focus particularly on evidence of my humanistic approach and she admitted that she had not considered this in her review. We were still able to discuss this aspect and I gave her several examples from my practice in the session and connected this to both my humanistic and andragogical underpinnings.

My reviewer and I disagreed on the level of my teacher competence using Benners' (1984) novice–expert scale. I felt that I had given a proficient demonstration of my teaching skills and that I had used theoretical constructs to guide, inform and change my action within the session; however, I had also noted some weaknesses in my performance. My reviewer insisted that I had given an expert demonstration, and although it was pleasing to be rated in this way, she was unable to justify why she had given such a high rating or give examples to support her judgement. She was likewise unable to suggest any areas of weakness in my teaching skills and knowledge which would help my future practice.

I have realised that it is very important for me that feedback, evaluation and assessment of my practice by self and others, continues to play a central role in my ongoing development. It is similarly important that in future I choose reviewers who are focused and knowledgeable about the areas of my practice which aid this development. The next time I am reviewed I am going to be much more explicit about the areas of the review which require detailed feedback and will also ensure that there is time allowed after the session for an immediate evaluation and reflective dialogue.

My experience of educational supervision began as an unqualified teacher and was closely related to ideas of mentorship, management and support in the workplace (Faugier 1992). There were other forms of supervision available to me on my teaching course, which centred around academic support and challenge and assessment roles and practice mentorship in terms of monitoring the competence of teaching practice. I found none of these roles and relationships wholly satisfactory and all of them inherently hierarchical. When I was asked by a colleague to be her educational supervisor I was unsure about both the nature of the role and, perhaps more importantly, my abilities to fulfil such a role.

I had an image of educational supervision as a possible vehicle for fostering reflective dialogue and practice among nurse educators, in part because I realised that this sort of relationship could have helped me foster my own reflective practice at a much earlier stage than I had reached it. I was also interested in the relationship from quite a selfish point of view and this reminded me of my days in clinical practice when I was the designated person who was interested in student mentorship. I always learned so much from my involvement in student learning and challenge to my own and others' practices. Supervision similarly offered both myself and the supervisee opportunities for continued development. I developed through my own negative and positive experiences of being supervised what my supervisor role might and has become. This final reflective excerpt unravels some of my thoughts and feelings about supervision and mentorship in nurse education.

The supervisor's story

From expert to novice and back again

When I was asked by a colleague to become her supervisor, I was unsure about the nature of the role and, perhaps more importantly, my abilities to fulfil such a role. I began by reading literature relating to supervision (Johns 1993; McIntyre *et al.* 1993, to name but a few), and this helped to clarify things somewhat. My experiences of supervision as a supervisee also influenced me and this combination of reading and experience shaped my expectations and ideas of what my role has become. I began to reflect on my knowledge and experience of supervision and the final two reflective extracts are significant in helping to unravel the process of becoming an effective and reflective supervisor.

As a student teacher, one of my supervisors adopted a parental, authoritative and supportive role. No formal contract was agreed between us, although we had decided on the timing, frequency and confidentiality of our supervisory sessions. The content of sessions invariably wandered off into chatting about colleagues or organisational issues which remained unresolved. Sometimes in sessions my supervisor would 'take over' and relate to me her own problems which remained unresolved. I felt relegated and reduced to the role of sympathiser and passive listener and found this devaluing and uncomfortable.

There was little or no challenge made to my own or the supervisor's educational practices, beliefs and values and I felt that we were getting nowhere. My own supervisor underrated and minimised the value of reflection and reflective teaching. Added to this, my supervisor regularly cancelled our sessions or the sessions were cut short or interrupted regularly. I felt that I didn't have her attention or interest when she was constantly looking at her watch. This experience led me to realise what I didn't want in a supervisory relationship and was positive in that I was able to uncover through reflection the sort of supervisor I would eventually become.

Another experience of supervision offered a more positive role model for my future supervisory role. In this relationship my supervisor constantly challenged my practice, beliefs and values. Her challenges, facilitated by reflective thinking, dialogue and actions, were to become the foundations on which my role as a supervisor evolved. Sessions were always dynamic and initially for me, uncomfortable, mainly because my habitual and unthinking practices were being exposed. I would go to her expecting her to offer advice, or to direct my thinking and actions, instead she refused to be prescriptive or solve my problems for me, which led to more confusion on my part.

On reflection I realised that she was practising the principles underpinning adult learning and education (Knowles 1978). Her skill as a supervisor, although unsettling for me, lay in her ability to help me develop my own decision-making abilities and resolve my own problems. Rather than telling me what to do, she would help me explore various options to test out in future practice. In retrospect this was crucial in developing my own reflective abilities and gave me the skills and knowledge with which I could continue to learn.

These experiences helped me to understand, develop and become more as a supervisor and teacher practitioner. I acknowledged my supervisee's need to perceive me as an 'expert' practitioner on which to base her 'novice' practices, and through reflective dialogue and writing we mutually explored these notions in a critical way. I noticed that within sessions there was often a conscious switching of my roles between critical friend, supporter, educator and facilitator as responses to the perceived needs of the supervisee, which Schön (1987) terms as, reflection in action. As the relationship evolved it became apparent to both of us that the central use of reflection in the supervisory process was effective and liberating for both of us.

Moreover, over a period of time it became obvious to both of us that the level of reflection we used had evolved and changed. Initially the supervisee highlighted basic questions about the nature and quality of her teaching work. Later in the relationship fundamental questions relating to the social and moral dimensions of the educational workplace were raised. This connects very well to Carr and Kemmis's (1986) work pertaining to the development of a:

> 'critical educational science [based on reflection which] has the aim of transforming education ... for students, teachers and society.' (Carr & Kemmis 1986, pp. 156–7)

To be effective supervision in an educational context needs to contain elements of guidance, support and challenge and more besides. Supervision can be practised as a learning experience and a relationship in which both parties are able to challenge and support their own and others' practices, values and beliefs, and even to challenge the supervisory relationship itself. The importance of challenge in the relationship is exemplified through my earlier reflections as a student teacher. Had I not received this challenge, it is doubtful that I would have been enabled to become insightful about my professional practice, or to have become reflective, or to have possessed the wherewithal to change and improve my practice. Challenge is essential within the relationship as it exposes and breaks down habitual practices (feelings, thoughts and actions). As Jarvis (1994) succinctly notes:

> 'People who know the truth are incapable of further learning.' (Jarvis 1994)

Although my supervisee initially saw me as an 'expert' practitioner on which to base her own 'novice' educational practice, I neither felt like or believed that I could fulfil this expectation. Moreover, I doubted her perception and self-proclaimed novice status. By exploring these issues through reflective dialogue in supervision, which consisted of mutual support, challenge and change followed by further reflection, the relationship moved beyond hierarchy and this was very liberating for both of us. I learned that sometimes the art of effective supervision lay in the non-intervention of the supervisor. The skill is deciding and intuitively knowing when to withdraw and facilitate the supervisee's decision-making processes; at other times it was appropriate to offer theoretical or experiential guidance and support.

My role as an educational supervisor has become redefined, the purposes of which are largely concerned with professional and personal development, of becoming more through reflection and reflective practice. My journey continues to unfold as I seek out other paths to walk along in equal partnership with those prepared to seek out other ways of knowing and being.

Conclusion

Throughout this chapter I have attempted to provide snapshots of my progression as a person and professional and some of the transformatory processes and outcomes of the development of my reflective activities. To some extent, although I have told my story in two halves, personal and professional transformation, for the purposes of providing a backdrop for professional transformation, the two are inextricably linked. Personal transformation and the development of reflectivity impact on professional activities, and similarly if one becomes reflective in professional life, this spills over and affects one's personal life.

I feel and hope that I have represented some of the significant moments in my life which led to my becoming reflective, and have shown why I continue to use reflection in personal and professional relationships to become more. Looking back on my experiences I recognise that reflection has opened up, and continues to open up, new possibilities of thinking, feeling and acting – the beginning of further development rather than the end of a particular problematic activity. Reflective practice indicates not the closure of a circle of thought, but a continuing spiral of possible other thoughts, other changes and other developments. My story is, therefore, incomplete. By articulating and sharing the changes and transformations that I have described, this makes the likelihood of new transformations and changes to future thinking and practices more possible. I am actively seeking other paths to walk down.

References

Benner, P. (1984) *From Novice to Expert: Excellence and Power in Clinical Nursing Practice*. Addison Wesley, Menlo Park, California.

Bernstein, B. (1975) *Class, Codes and Control*. Routledge and Kegan Paul, London.

Boud, D., Keogh, R. & Walker, D. (1985) (eds) *Reflection: Turning Experience into Learning*. Kogan Page, London.

Carr, W. & Kemmis, S. (1986) *Becoming Critical: Education, Knowledge and Action Research*. Falmer/Deakin University Press, Lewes.

Cohen, L. (1975) *Leonard Cohen: Greatest Hits*. C.B.S. Records.

Cohen, L. (1992) *The Future*. Sony Music Entertainment Inc.

Escher, M.C. (1989) *The Graphic Work*. Cordon Art. Baarn, Holland.

Faugier, J. (1992) The supervisory relationship. In *Clinical Supervision & Mentorship in Nursing* (T. Butterworth & J. Faugier). Chapman Hall, London.

Jarvis, P. (1994) *Lecture given at Institute for Nursing*. Radcliffe Infirmary, Oxford.

Johns, C.C. (1993) Professional supervision. *Journal of Nursing Management*, **1**(1), 9–18.

Knowles, M. (1978) *The Adult Learner: a Neglected Species?*, 2nd edn. Gulf Publishing, Houston.

McIntyre, D. Hagger, H. & Wilkin, D. (eds) (1993) *Mentoring Perspectives on School Based Teacher Education*. Kogan Page, London.

Paterson, J.G. & Zderad, L.T. (1976) *Humanistic Nursing*. John Wiley, New York.

Schön, D.A. (1987) *Educating the Reflective Practitioner*. Jossey Bass, San Francisco.

Chapter 17

The Rocky Road to Reflection

Myra Davis

Introduction

Many nurses remain sceptical about the potential of reflection to transform practice. This chapter aims to address some of the issues for qualified nurses, sometimes of many years' experience, who may see reflective practice as little more than a method of justifying our actions, rather than a way to relate theory to practice. It can be hard for a practitioner working in isolation to integrate appropriate nursing theory when the priority remains delivery of care quickly and within reduced resources. Equally it can be hard for the theorist to form relationships with practitioners who work to a very different agenda. I believe that the greatest strength of reflective practice is its ability to provide an opening from theory into practical implementation of what we know to be good nursing practice. My argument throughout this chapter will therefore be that reflective practice can provide us with the cornerstone of nursing practice, increase our self-confidence and allow us to begin to articulate what it is that a qualified nurse is best placed to do. Our inability to explain the role of the qualified nurse presents a challenge to the society of nursing, and our willingness to allow our role to be eroded constitutes an assault on what we expect of ourselves and what our patients are entitled to expect, and how they see and think of us.

My personal experience of growth is a key factor in my search for an enlightened way of caring, as I knew that to be clear in my own purpose is to be clear in the purpose of others. Coming to reflective practice purely by chance in October 1994, I found myself in a somewhat confused state. I was working as an ex-nurse manager and like many others was trying to find new ways of being in today's Health Service, an organisation I wanted to stay in and whose existence mattered to me very much. I and my colleagues found the culture to be changing so rapidly that to say, 'I've seen this idea before – it doesn't work', was easily translated into a resistance to change. This made me wary, unconfident and feeling that I could not say what I believed and how I felt in many situations. However, I felt I had something to contribute, and I wanted to find a way of ensuring that the experienced nurses I worked with continued to believe that expert nursing care was still the key to the patient's experience of healthcare.

I saw increasing distress and lack of confidence in ward sisters who were no longer able to trust their hearts to decide the best way to care for themselves, their patients and their staff. They felt the reason they were there – to provide clinical advice, excellence in patient care and effective role modelling for the future – was no longer the most important thing. There also appeared to be a feeling of isolation from the decision-making process, possibly due to a lack of support from nurse managers and an inability due to external constraints to deliver the type of care they wished. Schön (1987) identified this degree of isolation stating that:

> 'In the varied topography of professional practice, there is a hard, high ground overlooking a swamp. On the high ground, manageable problems lend themselves to solutions through application of research based theory and technique. In the swampy lowland, messy confusing problems defy technical solution. The irony of the situation is that the problems of the high ground tend to be relatively unimportant to individuals or society at large, whilst in the swamp lie the problems of greatest human concern.'

I realised strongly that I had to find some way of making sense of how my colleagues and myself were feeling, and find a way to move forward. For me, there was also an increasing anger that qualified nurses were either unable or unwilling to empower themselves, and appeared to have little knowledge of their experience, expertise and potential strength (Gibson 1991). This lack of perceived power often seemed to be based on an inability to forgive themselves for their lack of control of their clinical environments, thus creating feelings that they had failed as leaders.

But what is forgiveness? We give ourselves such a hard time for what we see as our failings and rarely recognise what we are good at. When the word forgiving is mentioned, what comes into your mind? Who is the person, or what is the experience you feel you will never forgive, never forget? When we refuse to forgive, we hold onto the past, and I know now that if you hold onto the past, you cannot live in the present. The concept of living in the present through forgiveness is addressed in Hay (1990). She states that:

> 'It is only when you are in the present that you can create your future. There is a tremendous sense of freedom that comes with forgiveness, and seeing the old pain and bitterness roll off your shoulders allows you to let go.' (p. 91)

Holding on to the past may have been an issue for these senior nurses as well. Was the old system really better, or did it often provide the comfort of a known routine? The effects of the health service reviews on staff have been widely researched. In 1993, after questioning nurses at ward sister level, McKenzie found that:

> '80% reported a belief in reinstating a purely nurse manager structure above G grade, 25% did not feel free to make autonomous decisions on clinical and professional matters, and 79.5% felt that the Health Service Reviews had a negative influence on their career directions.' (McKenzie 1993)

I wanted to find a way to help staff feel more confident and comfortable with today's health service, and I wanted to find a way for myself and for them of moving away from the need to justify, quantify and prove nursing actions and knowledge. Sometimes we did know what was the most appropriate action just because of the experience we had, and De Saint Exupery (1949) illustrated for me what was best about being a qualified nurse and what was easily identifiable in my colleagues, when he said:

> 'It is only with the heart that one can see rightly: what is essential is invisible to the eye.' (p. 70)

I believed that a way of achieving this was to look at mechanisms to increase the sense of who we are, creating a future that embraces our inherent rightness in our work.

Certain theorists remain for me key works for defining the nature and importance of my reflective practice needs, and as reflection provides a way of gaining professional and social awareness, these tend to be somewhat action based, describing the catalytic potential. Fay (1987) showed that learning through reflection is:

> 'Enlightenment   –   To understand who I am,
> Empowerment   –   To have the courage to change who I am, and
> Emancipation   –   To liberate myself to become who I need to be.'

I believe that the fundamental success of reflection for each individual must rest on their willingness to involve themselves in the development of self-insight and confidence, as a result leading to changed perspectives. It is these crucial aspects that distinguish reflection from analysis. Reflection as a learning tool is a necessary process for a professional to educate themselves, and if learning is to occur from practice, this period of personal examination and reconciliation is vital.

Transforming practice

When learning through group reflection I became involved on a weekly basis with a group of articulate supportive professionals who shared experiences of often frightening intensity. The sessions were led by an experienced facilitator and supervisor and formed part of the course on becoming a reflective practitioner.

I realised that often things were not what they seemed, and I began to see the nonsensical situation we have got ourselves into in clinical practice in that we need to name skills of nursing that do not need to be named, and often name them incorrectly, denying the importance of what they obviously are. I was recently teaching a group of health care assistants, and we discussed the subject of job satisfaction. Jane, an HCA of 18 months' experience who had not finished level 2 NVQ, told me that she was having a great time – Sister was teaching her to perform male and female catheterisation. When I recovered from my shock, I saw the relevant Sister in the corridor and I said, 'I understand you are teaching Jane to catheterise'. She was not surprised by my question. 'Oh yes,' she said. 'She's brilliant. I just set up the trolley, and when we are busy, off she goes.' 'So,' I replied, 'when you are admitted in retention of urine, you'll be happy for her to catheterise you, will you?' Without measuring her response at all, she said, 'Oh no, I'd want a qualified nurse'.

The experience in this story encapsulates nursing's difficulty in defining what it is that is so important for a qualified nurse to do. The image of nursing, cost constraints, resource issues and role conflicts have become muddled with what is tangible and real. We all believe that qualified nurses give the highest quality care.

As a result of these thoughts, I started to work with several senior nurses in different districts. At their request we started to examine incidents and issues in their practice to see if there were recognisable trends that may be addressed. Reflection was guided by a model I have used often, particularly with those less familiar with reflection who often feel safer with a structure in the early phase – that of Johns (1994), worked around Carper (1978).

Sarah

Sarah is a senior nurse who asked me to assist her with some interviews for new staff. I queried whether her manager knew she had asked me, and whether she was happy for me to be involved. She said she would not ask her; she believed her manager had no interest in what she did and only criticised her for any decisions she made herself. However, if she criticised any of her manager's views, she was told that if she didn't like it she could find a new job. The result of this breakdown in communication was that Sarah knew her credibility as a clinical manager was being affected as she did not feel able to lead.

Discussing this with Sarah, her main worry appeared to be her relationship with the team in the light of how they had seen her react to her manager, rather than the relationship with the manager itself. This often seemed to manifest as a need to be seen by the team as being bolder than her manager, whom she would abuse to the team after she had left the ward. Together we identified the key issues for Sarah. These included a need to feel that her manager respected her, for her team to know this, and she needed a sense of ownership of issues within her clinical area.

Meeting with her every two weeks, she shared reflection via the model. It became apparent that conflict and confrontation had happened with her previous manager, but her perception of this in relation to the current conflict was totally different; in many ways she found the old conflict stimulating and thought provoking. She did know sometimes that her previous manager was irritated with her, and as this happened so rarely it gave importance to the issue and made her choose to address it.

So we decided to examine a strategy by which Sarah would first feel confident to address issues with her manager, even if this invoked a negative response. This involved reflecting on clinical situations she had been involved in, and creating a sense of self-esteem as a clinical practitioner. By beginning to develop insight into the strength of her experience, we then moved on to methods she might feel able to adopt with her manager, all of which were suggested by herself. A great deal of this work was assisting her in reminding herself that she actually did know a great deal, and that the type of experience and knowledge she had was crucial to any decisions about her ward, her team or herself.

After we had met for several sessions, Sarah began to see that the confrontation was not her fault: that she had reacted negatively to her manager as she felt challenged. This struggle for power had meant that her manager had tried to dominate her, forcing her into confrontation and thus making her feel weaker as she built herself up to be combative before any interactions happened.

Sarah's work has proved to be worthwhile for us both, as I have begun to see the beginnings of a transformation. Sarah is beginning to find her strength, and she has said she does not have to justify herself so much with her team any more, as she feels more confident that they will realise she is a good sister without being influenced by her interactions with her manager. Her relationship in this area is still being addressed, but she appears less afraid of trying to start a conversation with her manager as her own self-esteem has begun to increase.

Sandy

Sandy is a senior nurse from a small unit who asked me to assist her with some work on skill mix. She had recently undertaken a skill mix review within her organisation without any training or knowledge of the implications, also under a very tight deadline. Completing the initial report, she was now being asked by her manager to extend the study into firm strategies to reduce the nursing budget. She compared this to being on a runaway train – she felt she had no control or direction. She knew the initial work she had undertaken resulted in a need to increase the skill mix, not reduce it, and felt if she assisted her manager in the strategy she would be seen to be reneging on her responsibilities as a ward leader to her staff. However, rather than discussing alternative approaches with her manager, she had decided that she would not do the work involved, as she was required to present a business plan to determine how she was going to carry out her manager's request. She had decided that her holding tactic, so she could avoid the stress of something she was not equipped to do, would be to tell her manager she was too busy, thus reassigning her agenda at ward level as more vital than that of the manager, falsely increasing her feelings of importance. When asked how she would feel if her manager then carried out the skills mix changes without her involvement, she stated that she would have to live with that, but it would not be her fault.

We discussed her need to confront her moral dilemma with her manager, and her need to discuss with the senior members of her team the pressure she was under, so they could form a strong group to give her support at this time of stress. She decided she needed to affirm her right to say no.

Meeting up with her some time later, I asked what had happened. Looking slightly bashful, she said she had decided to avoid the work, which had resulted in angry confrontations with her manager. Her manager, however, had not made the skill mix changes as a result, and Sandy felt this proved a justification for her course of action, and did not appear unduly concerned that she had maintained this way of acting. Overall, this was not a satisfactory conclusion but illustrated that practitioners who are not given regular support will often not address issues that may prove challenging, painful and uncomfortable. Not everyone feels able to reflect on practice and identify areas for transformation; others, when offered support, will seize the opportunity. For me, reflection has become part of my very existence; indeed, not so much an educator but a way of being. They are inextricably linked. I am reminded of the words of Aoki (1990):

> 'To me, an educated person, first and foremost, understands that one's ways of knowing, thinking and doing flow from who one is. Such a person knows that an authentic person is no mere individual, an island unto oneself, but is a being in relation with others, and hence, is at core, an ethical being. Moreover, a truly educated person speaks and acts from deep sense of humility, conscious of the limits set by human finitude and mortality, acknowledging the grace by which educator and educated are allowed to dwell in the present that embraces past experiences but is open to possibilities yet to be.' (p. 42)

I am willing to learn new things because I do not know it all. I am willing to drop old concepts when they no longer work for me. I am willing to see situations about myself and say, 'I don't want to do that any more'. I know I can become more of who I am. Not a better person, because that implies I am not good enough, but I can become more of who I am. Growing and chancing is exciting, even if I have to look at some painful things inside me to do it. I can see the possibilities for all of us, and that for me can be frustrating, because I know how strong we could be if only we believed it. This reflective practitioner needed to learn the skills of patience and the process of transformation. I feel reassured by the words of Emden (1991) who writes:

'The significance of how you approach your work and reframe its problems will quickly be noticed by those around you: a ripple effect becomes evident as others seek to understand and emulate your ideas and practices.'

Conclusion

It hasn't all been easy, though, and for a new student of reflective practice the writing available can be complex and confusing. To know that the reality of your practice lives up to your aspirations, you need to be confident that you have the theoretical background to assist you. Reflective theory could be equated with liquorice allsorts: you often don't know that a writer is not for you until you have tasted their work, and I have found I have had to reject many renowned writers on reflection, often due to their turgidity.

And I have found that many of the arguments against reflection have a clarity of thought and a critical approach that has often made me return to my philosophy and check that it still suits me. Reflection is an impressive tool. It has the power and immediacy to astonish the practitioner as it brings about revolutions in their practice, and the understanding that comes through close examination of feelings and actions allows the most powerful experiences to be put into perspective. This does, however, involve a great deal of letting go – letting go of thoughts, rationalisations and of knowing. In *Glimpse after Glimpse*, Rinpoche (1995) suggests that although our minds are wonderful, they can be at the same time our very worst enemy. When we begin to experience our knowing from a peace inside, it is not instead of or as a substitute for the mind's knowing, it is as well as – a complementary knowing. Becoming and remaining a good nurse is relentless unending work. Demonstrating the commitment to grow and develop via reflective practice is often painful, but can give moments of insight that give great joy and contribute to a personal strength that lends itself to growth in all aspects of an individual's being. Knowing that you need to keep at it means that enquiry is usually at the forefront of your mind: Why is this happening? What part do I play? How should I act?

We all know nurses who are party to stupid, unexplainable actions that they then justify by saying, 'But what could I do?'. I know now that this will not do for me anymore. Emden (1991) in discussing the difficulties of writing, said:

'On becoming reflective, the compulsion to address issues is the same: all mental rooms are cleansed and a new way of being is found.'

References

Aoki, T. (1990) Inspiring the curriculum. *The ATA Magazine*, Jan/Feb, p. 37–42.

Carper, B. (1978) Fundamental patterns of knowing in nursing advances. *Nursing Science*, 1, 13–23.

De Saint Exupery, A. (1949) *The Little Prince*. Piccolo, London.

Emden, C. (1991) Becoming a reflective practitioner. In *Towards a Discipline for Nursing*. Churchill Livingstone, London.

Fay, B. (1987) *Critical Social Science*. Polity Press, Cambridge.

Gibson, C. (1991) A concept analysis of empowerment. *Journal of Advanced Nursing*, 16, 354–61.

Hay, L. (1990) *Heart Thoughts*. Airlift Book Company, Enfield, Middlesex.

Johns, C. (1994) *Model of Structured Reflection*, 10th edn. Faculty of Health and Social Studies, University of Luton.

McKenkie, J. (1993) Effects of change on ward sisters and charge nurses. *Nursing Standard*, 7(36), 25–7.

Rinpoche, S. (1995) *Glimpse After Glimpse*. Random House, London.

Schön, D. (1987) *Educating the Reflective Practitioner*. Jossey Bass, London.

Chapter 18
A Meta-reflection on Reflective Practice and Caring Theory

Jean Watson

Introduction

Reflective practice, at its most basic core, is about 'seeing' and uncovering nursing at its core. In so doing, it has evolved from a critical model of scholarship, which critiques any dominant discourse or overlay of theory. This process of uncovering new meanings 'from the ground up', in contrast to 'seeing' from the 'top down' through the lens of discipline defining theory, creates an inherent dissonance between the latest developments in reflective practice and the movement to theory guided practice as a means of demonstrating nursing's unique approach to both knowledge and practice. This tension has been labelled by Schön (1987) as the high ground of abstract theory which often stands in sharp contrast to the lowlands, the marsh, the mysterious, dark day to day world which often defies abstract solutions.

This high ground/lowland – mountain/marsh topography of nursing science is part of the most contemporary modern-postmodern debate and discourse in science itself. That is, we are at somewhat of a cross-roads between centuries, world views, paradigms and research traditions, whereby new questions are being asked and new challenges are being faced about these differences.

Critics in all fields acknowledge that the empirical-analytic model of science has allowed the physical-material-objectivist knowledge to take precedence over any other knowledge. The disownment of any grand theory from the mountain, which may totalise the discourse and rule out other ways of seeing from the marsh, has become the rule in the post-modern critiques of knowledge, theory and science itself.

The reflective practice momentum in the UK, and to some extent in Australia and New Zealand, represents the marsh end of the spectrum with respect to nursing science and uncovering new knowledge of practice. Whereas the US and Canada seem to represent the mountain end of the debate with respect to nursing knowledge development.

So, then, where does theory fit within this reflective practice movement, or does it? One argument is that it is through nursing theory that nursing determines (or constructs) its field of knowledge. Hence, the classic statement of Carper has often been cited to make the case for theory guided practice:

'It is the general conception of any field of inquiry that ultimately determines the kind of knowledge the field aims to develop, as well as the manner in which that knowledge is to be organized, tested, and applied.' (1978, p. 13)

More recently, Reed (1995, p. 76) noted that it is through the '... values initially put forth by modernist nursing, that distinguish nursing knowledge and the caring application of that knowledge'.

In spite of that position with respect to nursing's field of knowledge, when one works 'from the ground up' in reflective practice models, a case comes to be made for practice guided theory as the basis for determining nursing's field of knowledge. When considering reflective practice perspective, the equation is turned around.

It seems that we can and do get caught in the middle of this modern, postmodern debate. It is true that while we can admit that the old story will no longer hold about totalising theory, the new story of science is not yet in place (Marcus 1994). We are still wandering without a clear direction somewhere between the mountain and the marsh. We are each trying to chart our way but in different terrain, of which the geography at either altitude is not clear and is constantly changing. Perhaps it is on occasions where we can reconsider theory and reflective practice activities at a meta-reflective level that we may see some common ground, that might unite the mountain and marsh, allowing for a new landscape for nursing science.

What has evolved to date, from both the lowlands dark view, and the cloudy, misty mountain view, is uncharted territory in which everything we thought we knew or could see is being dismantled all around us. In this free-floating, constantly changing space, we have arrived at a place of unending relativism, existential finitude, unravelling of reality, scientific and social confusion, human and environmental violence and even a sense of moral anarchy. In this postmodern space where nursing science and all sciences now float, we ponder the possibility that even humanity and the planet itself cannot hold (Lather 1991).

Both mountain-marsh positions seem to be held in somewhat of a juxtapositional limbo at this turn in the modern-postmodern developments in nursing, and in other sciences. This modern-postmodern crisis in science and method is now part of the landscape and backdrop for considering the role of caring theory and reflective practice.

While the two positions seem to stand in opposition to each other and be radically diametric in their perspective, there is another position that is emerging which helps to integrate the two opposites. After a couple of decades of deconstructing the knowledge-power-politics nexus of both theory and science, there is an ironic return to grand theory in the human sciences (Skinner 1994). This turn has implications for reflective practice activities and offers a new clearing whereby the mountain and marsh can converge, but for different reasons that originally posited in the postmodern discourse.

In this one moment in history we are in the position of disowning any theory or method, or any dominating system, while paradoxically needing some lens through which to reflect upon what we are seeing; indeed, we seem to be in need of a lens 'to see' before we can even reflect upon what has taken place in a given moment. Or to put it another way, if you cannot 'see' differently, you cannot act differently. As my colleague and friend Luther Christman put it years ago: 'You can't use knowledge you don't have'.

Using caring theory as a lens for 'reflective seeing' helps to bring the mountain and marsh closer together to create a new territory. This integration of the two can offer nursing knowledge that can be used to both inform and transform practice. To begin with, in a return to grand theory, we find that the Greek word for theory comes from the word 'theoria', meaning 'to see'. Reflective practice, as already noted, is also about 'seeing'. From that starting point alone, one can see the common quests in the two endeavours, moving to the notion of 'reflective seeing'. In reconsidering caring theory as a reflective lens, it has ontological and epistemological implications for practice and for approaches toward inquiry. Caring theory at the macro level can be considered a philosophy, an ethic, an ethos and part of the evolving paradigm for the entire discipline.

Using this as a lens for reflective practice and social action research, one can seek to uncover the many aspects of caring and the many diverse ways that it manifests itself in the nurse–person caring relationship; e.g. a human trait, a moral imperative, an effect, an interpersonal interaction, a therapeutic intervention and so on (Morse *et al.* 1991).

When caring theory is introduced to reflective practice initiatives, it becomes part of the dialogue which seeks to reconcile a basic awareness about the relational values and beliefs nursing holds (Reed 1995), for example, unity of mind, body and spirit, wholeness and healing and the interplay between the objective and subjective worlds of human experiences. This lens stands in contrast to an objectivist curing lens, looking for physical diagnosis and treatment. In other words, caring theory with its explicit philosophy of an ethic of caring, context and meaning, along with its set of embedded values toward person, unity of being, relation and so on, serves as a meta-lens for reflecting/re-reflecting, re-visioning nursing practice.

Nursing scholars in the area of reflective practice inquiry could then look through this meta-lens to form their critique of practice knowledge and how caring and wholeness, for example, manifests (or does not manifest) in action. It is here that nursing rsearch stimulates greater awareness and creative scholarship, inquiring about caring processes ranging from systems of care to human caring processes, relationships, aspects of intuition and presence, all the way to advanced caring–healing modalities and advanced nursing caring therapeutics.

Reflective practice models guided by caring theory lens

This perspective on caring as a meta-lens for reflective practice inquiry leads to other developments and the emergence of new models that are actually transformative. Indeed, if one is truly committed to transforming nursing, to be more consonant with its values and philosophies of caring, some deeper insight is called for.

Reflective caring practice models seeking true transformation will evolve to include a deeper way of obtaining insight as a way of both seeing and being. For example, one insight that comes from reflective practice momentum is a 'return to the things themselves' as the basis for seeing. In this new landscape being created we have to go to the territory itself. However, in this territory we can seek the treasures in the boggy marsh, by exploring each caring occasion, by honouring and honing each caring moment as a moment of possibility for learning about wholeness of being. In these moments we can uncover the artistry of the caring-healing practices.

Reflective caring practice is first of all related to Hannah Arendt's pleas to 'stop and think' (Arendt 1961). By that, reflective caring practice helps us to stop and pause in the midst of action. To be more aware, more mindfully, authentically present, allowing a re-direction, or re-reflection in the midst of action, without interrupting it. This may be as simple as shifting one's consciousness from being harried, hurried or rushed, to being still, to find one's quiet centre, in the midst of the act, and hold such a conscious quiet stillness toward self and other.

The reflection practice research models in the UK use the term supervision as part of the reflective process of inquiry. In uniting caring with reflective practice research, we may choose to reconsider that term. Through reflective caring practices we allow ourselves to step back, observe and reflect upon our acts and actions, to describe, connect with them at a deeper level of 'seeing', to search for Polanyi's tacit knowing (Polanyi 1964). In this process of mutuality with another we are invited to draw upon intuition, to unravel the moment and learn from it, to make explicit, symbolic, even metaphorical, something that was implicit, tacit and spontaneous, but nevertheless was a knowledgeable action, capable of knowing and learning about at a deeper level.

This form of supervision, which assists others in 'seeing through the glass darkly', can be re-framed as coaching, mentoring, or opportunities for genuine dialogue, rather than supervision in the conventional modern sense of the word. Through such a supportive process, the evolved method thus becomes one of reflective caring inquiry. In this kind of inquiry, that which was uncovered in the bog can serve as a new lens by which to 'see' next time. This developed conscious-intentional reflection-in-action can serve to reshape what we are doing while we are doing it.

This process gives rise to what Mary Catherine Bateson called prac-tised improvisation (Bateson 1990), whereby each caring moment, each caring occasion, presents a new moment of possibility for both the nurse and the one being cared for; how to consider being in the moment; each moment a unique, not repeatable instance, an opportunity for better improvising for full use of self and relational caring competencies to be more fully actualised.

Such informed reflective caring practice becomes artful use of self, requiring artistry for each occasion of being human, calling upon all ways of knowing in one act. Some indicate that 'seeing' cannot be taught; it must be witnessed and experienced for self, which requires coaching.

Some artful caring practice can also be learned through story-telling, poetry, film, artwork, literature, drama – all of which reveal a 'right kind of truth telling', a deep inner life world of knowing, that cannot be learned from the outer world alone (Noddings 1984).

In this new world of reflective caring practice and inquiry which is evolving, communities of practitioners can and are beginning to assist each other in responding to those indeterminate zones of mystery in their practice; they are providing each other with a reflective con-versation about a situation. Such communities of practitioners are making it possible to re-make a part of the practice world, and reveal the caring processes that underlie the daily work or reveal the obstacles to that process.

Clinical caritas: re-visioning reflective caring practice

Lastly, in the re-visioned reflective caring practice model, which allows the caring theory from the mountain to intersect and merge with the marsh, we can introduce the relationship between caring and love. By introducing the word love, we can explore the concept of clinical caritas. Caritas, related to the words charity, caring and cherish, is a Latin word meaning regard, affection, esteem and love, and also has the connotation of preciousness (Noddings 1984). It is also to be noted that the word 'carative' in caring theory (Watson 1979, 1985, 1988) is closely related to the Latin word caritas.

I admit, it is not popular or acceptable in traditional circles of nursing science and professional practice, to speak of love. Noddings & Shore (1984 p. 157) quote P.A. Sorokin who reminded us of this fact:

'The sensate minds, our minds, disbelieve the power of love. It appears to us illusionary – we call it self-deception; the opiate of a people's mind, idealistic thought and unscientific illusion.

We are biased against all theories that try to prove the power of love and other positive forces in determining human behavior and personality, in influencing the course of biological, social, moral, and mental evolution, in affecting the direction of historical events, in shaping social institutions and cultures.'

Others, such as Noddings, are in distinct opposition to such a denial of love's existence. When we introduce clinical caritas into our thinking in both education and practice, it becomes something very real. As an educator and philosopher, Noddings acknowledges love is a force that can be the most powerful agent in the classroom and leave the most lasting impressions, touch lives most deeply. By the concept of clinical or educational caritas, it is a desire to come into direct undiluted contact with the human dimensions of the other, to go beyond the superficialities and be engaged with the whole person (Noddings 1984).

Clinical caritas may also involve a deep interest and even passionate commitment to one's subject matter or the subjective life world of understanding the other and their concerns. Love as the core of clinical caritas is the source, the energy that provides the excitement, hope, passion, compassion needed to sustain caring relationships in the stultifying routines found in our institutions. The other facet of clinical caritas is a sense of what might even be called a mission, or a 'calling', that both nurses and educators have felt down through the ages. They know and experience the meaningfulness and rewards of human serving and contributing to the healing and growth of self and others. It is caritas which is the reason that teaching and practice are so often more than simply a job, and is an exhilarating, if challenging, experience, providing a foundation for a lifetime career (Noddings & Shore 1984).

Conclusion

In the end, when reflective caring practice activities and new communities of informed practitioners assert such concepts as love and caritas into their ways of being and knowing, then clinical caring processes will be turned into a sacred act. Nursing will then be able to cultivate a sense of 'sacred seeing', whereby it restores its very heart and soul.

Reflective caring practice and inquiry in a transformed model of clinical caritas become an occasion for learning, growing and practising, an occasion for being open to giving and receiving, to experience the mystery, the wonder, the whole of caring practices. Clinical caritas returns us to the true core of nursing, emerging with a new identity and renewed energy to come into our own, and open to our own awakening. Together we then enter a new land for post-postmodern nursing where caring theory and reflective practice are one.

References

Arendt, H. (1961) *Between Past and Future*. Viking, New York.

Bateson, M.C. (1990) *Composing a Life*. Plume, New York.

Carper, B. (1978) Fundamental patterns of knowing in nursing. *Advances in Nursing Science*, **1**(1), 13–23.

Lather, P. (1991) *Getting Smart*. Routledge, New York.

Marcus, G.E. (1994) What comes (just) after 'post'? In *Handbook of Qualitative Research* (eds N.K. Denzin & Y.S. Lincoln), pp. 563–74. Sage Publications, London.

Morse, J. Bottoroff, J., Neander, W. & Solberg, S. (1991) Comparative analysis of conceptualizations and theories of caring. *Image: The Journal of Nursing Scholarship*, **23**(2), 119–26.

Noddings, N. (1984) *Caring: A Feminine Approach to Ethics and Moral Education*. University of California Press, Berkeley.

Noddings, N. & Shore, P.J. (1984) *Awakening the Inner Eye*. N.Y. Teacher's College, Columbia University Press.

Polanyi, M. (1964) *Personal Knowledge: Towards a Post-Critical Philosophy*. Harper & Row, New York.

Reed, P.G. (1995) A treatise on nursing knowledge development for the 21st century: beyond postmodernism. *Advances in Nursing Science*, **17**(30) 70–84.

Schön, D. (1987) *Educating the Reflective Practitioner*. Jossey-Bass Publishers, San Francisco.

Skinner, Q. (ed) (1994) *The Return of Grand Theory in the Human Sciences*. Cambridge University Press, Cambridge.

Watson, J. (1979) *Nursing: the Philosophy and Science of Caring*. Little Brown, Boston. Reprinted in 1985 by Colorado Associated University Press.

Watson, J. (1985) *Nursing: Human Science and Human Care. A theory of nursing*. Appleton-Century-Crofts, Norwalk, CT.

Watson, J. (1988) *Nursing: Human Science and Human Care*. National League for Nursing, New York.

Index

alchemy, 17, 177

Burford NDU Model, 14–15,
        107–11, 116

clinical supervision, 7, 12–14,
        63–77, 104–16
critical social science, 77–8

empathy, 7
empowerment, 16, 18, 51–2
ethical mapping, 8
ethical reasoning, 9
evidence-based practice, 30
expanded consciousness, 6, 18, 51,
        54, 60, 89, 182

intuition, 1–3, 21–9

knowledge
    constructed, 58–9
    critical, 135–7
    empirical, 5–7, 29, 47, 135–6
    epistemology, 135, 216
    ethical, 5–7, 32–41, 47
    experiential, 22–3, 29
    expert, 1–3, 22–8
    interpretive, 135
    intuitive, 55
    personal, 5–7, 37–8, 47
    procedural, 57
    received, 54–5, 179

subjective, 55–6
tacit, 1–2, 22, 45, 183, 217

morality
    customary, 32–41
    reflective, 32–41
mythology, 177

nurse
    as artist, 47
    as assertive, 12, 60
    as caring, 43–7, 161–74
    autonomy, 34, 72
    humanistic existentialists, 153–5
    moral agent, 34–5
nursing
    actual practice, 9, 16
    advocacy, 127
    as profane, 17
    as sacred, 17
    care planning, 106
    clinical caritas, 13, 174, 218–19
    desirable practice, 9, 16, 64
    nursing process, 1, 104, 107
    philosophy, 63
    power, 12
    primary nursing, 107
    professional practice, 32–8

ontology, 135, 161–74, 216

personhood, 44–5

Pysche, 178

reflection
  as narrative, 15
  as research tool, 93
  as storytelling, 4, 43, 47–9, 95,
    98–102
  contradiction, 9–10, 17, 63, 79
  critical, 36, 94–102, 134, 138,
    143–7, 151, 157
  guided, 12–16, 60, 62–77, 80–89,
    112
  heuristic device, 3
  in action, 3, 14, 21–8, 45–6, 92,
    138, 151–2, 183
  interpretive reflection, 134,
    139–47, 165–74
  meta-reflection, 214
  model-structured reflection,
    3–11, 69, 112
  on action, 21–8, 64, 92, 138, 152,
    183
  on experience, 3, 14–15, 78–80
  phenomenological reflection,
    120–33

religion, 186–8
research
  action, 13, 28, 104–16
  case studies, 99
  collaborative, 120
  empirical, 165–6
  grounded theory, 4, 137
  phenomenology, 15–16, 137,
    139–43, 145–7
  triangulation, 166

self
  higher self, 17, 182–3
  knowing self, 16, 87–9
  spiritual self, 17, 188–92
suffering, 161–74, 177–8

theory
  extant, 10
  critical, 143
  personal, 28–9
therapeutic touch, 190
transformation, 10, 13, 18, 177
  through voice, 51–60